Cholesterol and Saturated Fat Prevent Heart Disease

Evidence From 101 Scientific Papers

By David Evans

Grosvenor House
Publishing Limited

This book is published by
Grosvenor House Publishing Ltd
28-30 High Street, Guildford, Surrey, GU1 3EL.
www.grosvenorhousepublishing.co.uk

A CIP record for this book
is available from the British Library

ISBN 978-1-78148-508-8

This book is dedicated to my father

Medical liability disclaimer

This book is intended solely for informational and educational purposes and not as medical advice, nor to replace the advice of a doctor or other health care professional. Anyone wishing to embark on any dietary or lifestyle change must first consult with his or her health care professional.

The decision to use any information in this book is entirely the decision of the reader, who assumes full responsibility for any and all consequences arising from such a decision. Neither the author nor the publisher shall be held liable for any consequences resulting or allegedly resulting from use of information in this book.

Table of contents

Introduction

This book is based on the findings of papers published in peer reviewed scientific journals, although the title does sound like something from a fantastic fairy tale. I mean "everybody knows" that cholesterol and saturated fat are the "twin evils" that lead to heart disease and an early death.

We have all heard that the standard dietary advice to prevent heart disease is to *cut right down* on cholesterol, red meat and saturated fats. To accompany this we are told we must eat plenty of carbohydrate rich, starchy foods such as bread, rice, potatoes and pasta. Again "everybody knows" this advice must be good for us.

Now imagine if what "everybody knows" is not true.

Imagine the dietary advice we have been given over the last four or five decades has been wrong.

Imagine the dietary advice we have been given actually contributes to the epidemics of heart disease, cancer, diabetes and neurological disorders.

I used to 100% believe that dietary cholesterol and saturated fat should be avoided and low fat diets should be embraced for the avoidance of heart disease and other conditions.

However over the years a few health problems started to appear. I had a nagging rash that would not clear up, and also suffered from athlete's foot. Regular bouts of heartburn used to punctuate my day and depressive episodes were beginning to blight my life. I was possibly pre-diabetic and my weight inexorably kept creeping up, to the point where I was thoroughly ashamed and embarrassed about myself.

Therefore I tried to lose weight by various means, the low fat route, the low calorie route and the extreme exercise route, but I always ended up eventually gaining extra weight.

A number of people I know started to suffer from cardiovascular diseases, cancer and other health problems, this at a relatively young age and despite them "taking their tablets" and adhering to a no smoking, low alcohol, low fat diet, moderate exercise type of lifestyle.

Nationally also, the incidence of these problems seems to increase inexorably.

For years I had an uneasy vague feeling that something must have changed, because many diseases and conditions that were rare or almost unheard of in previous generations were now commonplace.

This uneasy feeling (and my increasing girth) motivated me into nutritional research. I've literally read dozens of books and thousands of papers published in peer reviewed scientific journals on the subject of nutrition and health.

The result of this research manifests itself in the 101 scientific papers in this book. I personally applied the principles of this research and effortlessly lost over 50lb excess weight and my health problems disappeared without having to resort to medical treatment. My energy levels have surged, I feel more alive and I have an enhanced sense of well–being.

The knowledge I have gained from all this research has led me to believe the *eat low fat dietary mantra* is sadly misguided and in fact is a major cause in the rise of many health conditions, diseases and obesity.

Another apparently set in stone mantra is that high blood cholesterol levels will be the precursor to certain heart disease and an early death. This is another in the "everybody knows" category.

We are frequently encouraged to have our "cholesterol numbers checked" and almost invariably after the numbers have been analysed, we are advised they are high, so we are at risk of heart disease, and that we need to take a little pill called a statin to save our lives.

Research of the scientific literature regarding high cholesterol and disease reveals a completely different story.

High cholesterol levels are actually associated with a longer life, so by being prescribed cholesterol-lowering medication you are taking steps to shorten your lifespan.

Saturated fat and cholesterol are in fact essential for good health.

- More than half the brain is fat and cholesterol and over half that fat is saturated.
- Fat and cholesterol are major components of the myelin sheath that protects nerve fibres.
- Saturated fats are a rich source of the vitamins A, D and K2.
- They are the preferred fuel for the heart.
- They constitute more than half of the cell membrane.
- They are critical for healthy bones.
- They can reverse liver damage.
- They help to create a strong immune system.
- Cholesterol is essential for the production of hormones such as testosterone and oestrogen.
- Cholesterol is the precursor to vitamin D.
- Cholesterol acts as an antioxidant.
- It is needed for the brain to function properly.

As you can see saturated fat and cholesterol are vital nutrients.

You are probably wondering how we got to the state of affairs where we are told to abstain from foods that have nourished us for over $2^1/_2$ million years, to now be advised to consume a diet that is foreign to our body, and that we must take pills that reduce an essential nutrient.

This book will answer that question and more. You will see the evidence from 101 scientific papers, which show how the saturated fat/cholesterol/heart disease hypothesis was born, and despite billions of dollars and decades of research, the hypothesis has never been proven.

You will discover that high cholesterol actually prolongs life, and find out the real reasons why people may get heart disease.

Finally insights and observations are gleaned from eminent professors and doctors into why the saturated fat/cholesterol/heart disease hypothesis is false.

This book has been written for people who are worried about the health of their heart. The general public and health practitioners are probably unaware of some or even most of the information and evidence presented in this book.

This information and evidence, taken directly from the actual scientific papers on the subject of the causes and prevention of heart disease, will allow you and your doctor to make informed decisions on the best way to maintain and improve your heart health, without the need to rely on the erratic "everybody knows" method of healthy living.

How to use this book

This book contains 101 scientific papers which have virtually all been published in peer reviewed scientific journals.

The format of the book has been designed so you can analyse each paper independently, although you could read the whole book through, or pick a chapter where you need particular knowledge.

Every paper has a heading that gives the essence of its findings. Each paper also contains the name of the author, the title of the paper and where it was published.

I then try and describe the findings of the paper in a concise, easy to read manner. However some unfamiliar words are in the text, which are explained in the glossary.

For an example of the layout, paper 28 is shown below:

Paper 28
High fat diet reduces heart disease
risk and helps in weight loss
Foster GD et al A Randomized Trial of a Low-Carbohydrate Diet for Obesity. *New England Journal of Medicine.* Volume 348 : 2082-2090 May 22, 2003 Number 21

The paper heading is: "High fat diet reduces heart disease risk and helps in weight loss".

G D Foster was the author. (et al means "with others"). So other people also contributed to the paper.

The title of the paper is "A Randomized Trial of a Low-Carbohydrate Diet for Obesity"

It was published in the *New England Journal of Medicine*.

The date, volume and page numbers etc. of this paper is Volume 348 : 2082-2090 May 22, 2003 Number 21.

You may be wondering what peer reviewed scientific journals are.

Peer Review is a process that journals use to ensure the articles they publish represent the best scholarship currently available. When an article is submitted to a peer reviewed journal, the editors send it out to other scholars in the same field (the author's peers) to get their opinion on the quality of the scholarship, its relevance to the field, its appropriateness for the journal, etc. If these "peers" find the proposed article does not meet these rigorous standards then the article is rejected. This process is in stark contrast to the articles written in newspapers, which are based on circulation figures and personal opinions.

CHAPTER 1

It's never been proved that high cholesterol causes heart disease

The cholesterol/saturated fat/heart disease hypothesis is based on the theory that dietary cholesterol and dietary saturated fat raise the blood cholesterol levels which then "clog" the arteries, which progresses to heart disease.

How did this theory evolve? The following three papers describe the seminal experiments and studies on which the whole hypothesis hangs.

Paper 1
Rabbits and cholesterol

Bailey CH Atheroma and other lesions produced in rabbits by cholesterol feeding. *Journal of Experimental Medicine.* 1916 Jan 1; 23(1) : 69-84

Bailey reviewed papers from Ignatovski, Anitschkov (sometimes spelled Anichkov) and others regarding the theory that cholesterol fed to rabbits then developed into cholesterol rich deposits in the arteries.

Bailey did find that cholesterol fed rabbits went on to develop abundant deposits of cholesterol in their arteries.

These studies of rabbits (and other herbivorous animals) have since been cited as evidence of the cholesterol/heart disease hypothesis; namely that as cholesterol and fatty diets cause a build up of cholesterol in rabbits - therefore it must be the same in humans.

This evidence has been analysed by Dr Uffe Ravnskov, (a leading expert on cholesterol and heart disease), who noted the following flaws in the logic of extrapolating results from rabbit experiments to "real life" in humans.

- The rabbit is a vegetarian. It cannot digest or metabolize cholesterol.
- If a rabbit is forced to eat food it cannot digest or metabolize, then its blood cholesterol rises 10 to 20 times higher than the highest values ever noted in human beings.
- Unlike humans, cholesterol percolates all through the rabbit; its liver and kidneys become fatty. Its fur falls out, and its eyes become yellow from a build-up of cholesterol that it can neither store nor metabolize nor excrete.
- Finally it dies, not from heart disease but from loss of appetite and emaciation - it starves.
- The most striking fact is that it is impossible to induce a heart attack in a rabbit by dietary means alone.

In rabbits, cholesterol consumption causes a massive increase in blood cholesterol levels, whereas in most humans excessive cholesterol consumption does not cause any rise in blood cholesterol levels, and in the few humans that it does cause a very small rise there is NO increase in heart disease risk (*see paper 16*). Yet these early studies on rabbits are often quoted as testament that cholesterol and saturated fat cause heart disease in humans.

Paper 2
Ancel Keys 6 countries study actually shows the more animal fat and animal protein you eat, the longer you live!

Keys A Atherosclerosis: a problem in newer public health. *Journal of the Mount Sinai Hospital, New York.* 1953 Jul-Aug; 20(2) : 118-39

This study examined the effect of fat consumption and death rates from heart disease in males aged 55-59 from six countries.

In this study Keys (a researcher who had made his mind up without any scientific evidence that fat consumption was the cause of heart disease) set out to prove that a higher fat intake was associated with a higher death rate from heart disease.

He used data from six countries (Japan, Italy, United Kingdom, Australia, Canada and USA) that did seem to show that a higher fat consumption would lead to higher rates of heart disease.

However Keys actually had data for 22 countries. For reasons known only to him he decided to ignore the data from the other 16. The other countries were Austria, Ceylon, Chile, Denmark, Finland, France, Germany, Ireland, Israel, Mexico, Netherlands, New Zealand, Norway, Portugal, Sweden and Switzerland.

When the data for all 22 countries are taken into account, there is a totally different outcome.

The data actually shows:

- Those that ate more animal fat lived longer.
- Those that ate more animal protein lived longer.
- Those that ate more plant protein died earlier.
- Those that ate more carbohydrate died earlier.

This study from Keys is often quoted as proof that a high fat diet is dangerous. When Keys data is analysed it shows that more animal fat in the diet actually extends life, and more carbohydrate in the diet lowers life expectancy.

Paper 3
If he'd wanted, Ancel Keys could have proved that saturated fat gives protection from heart disease

Keys A Coronary heart disease in
seven countries. Summary. *Circulation.*
1970 Apr; 41(4 Suppl) : I186-95.

This study was designed by Ancel Keys to prove that a high saturated fat and high cholesterol consumption would lead to high rates of heart disease. It is possibly the single most important piece of research in the development of the saturated fat/cholesterol/heart disease hypothesis.

The study compared the rates of heart disease and saturated fat content in the diets of people from seven countries. The study was launched in 1958.

Keys chose the data from seven countries Italy, Greece, Former Yugoslavia, Netherlands, Finland, Japan and U.S.A. This data shows there is a correlation between saturated fat intake and heart disease. The study also claimed a link between higher cholesterol levels and heart disease.

However Malcolm Kendrick, a Scottish doctor and general practitioner for over 25 years who has also worked with the European Society of Cardiology, found if Keys had chosen to study seven other countries, Finland, Israel, Netherlands, Germany, Switzerland, France and Sweden, then he would have discovered the exact opposite. Namely, the more cholesterol/saturated fat consumed, the less heart disease.

Kendrick adds if you were to have chosen any other seven countries in the world, apart from the ones Ancel Keys chose, you would get a different set of results. A clue to how Keys came to choose his seven countries is given below.

Dr Kendrick also notes that as a piece of scientific research, the possibility that Ancel Keys introduced bias is so great that–were this study to be proposed today–it would be thrown out by any decent research committee.

This begs the question: Why did Keys manipulate the data?

One of Keys friends, Henry Blackburn, describes how Keys was previously humiliated about his saturated-fat/heart disease hypothesis *(see paper 2)* in a meeting called by the World Health Organisation in Geneva to discuss the rising rates of heart disease.

Keys was a very strong willed character, with a strong personality. He was quick to verbally attack anyone with whom he disagreed in an abusive scolding manner in both medical journals, and in person during conferences.

Blackburn's theory is that the humiliation at the World Health Organisation meeting was such that Keys was stung into action and was driven to find "evidence" to "prove" his saturated-fat/heart disease hypothesis-hence the seven countries study.

The preceding three papers show how the diet/ heart hypothesis is based on flawed experiments with herbivorous animals and extremely biased studies conducted by a man with "a chip on his shoulder". It's staggering and disturbing how the dietary advice for heart disease invariably given out by various governments around the world is based on these flawed papers.

The next five papers are all studies on the relationship of blood cholesterol levels and evidence of heart disease. The present day health authorities should take note of the results of these studies as they all come to the same conclusion-the level of the cholesterol in the blood has no association with the incidence of heart disease.

Paper 4
Harvard pathologist finds that high blood cholesterol is NOT the cause of blocked arteries
Lande KE, Sperry WM. Human atherosclerosis in relation to the cholesterol content of the blood serum.
Archives of Pathology. 1936; 22 : 301-312

In 1936, the pathologist Dr Kurt Lande and the biochemist Dr Warren Sperry at the department of Forensic medicine of New York University measured cholesterol levels and the deposition of fat in the aorta in people who had died sudden deaths.

They found there is no correlation between levels of cholesterol in the blood and the amount of blockage in the arteries. Some subjects had very low levels of cholesterol but a high amount of blockage, while others had high levels of cholesterol and a low amount of blockage.

Paper 5
Research team reveal cholesterol levels have NO correlation with clogged arteries

Mathur KS et al Serum cholesterol and
atherosclerosis in man. *Circulation.*
1961; 23 : 847-852

Two hundred cases of sudden death were selected from autopsies at the Sarojini Naidu Hospital, India by Dr Mathur and his research team for a study of the relationship of cholesterol levels to the amount and severity of clogged arteries in the aorta and the coronary and cerebral arteries.

The study found that no correlation could be observed between cholesterol levels and the amount and severity of clogged arteries.

Paper 6
The cholesterol/heart disease hypothesis is false

Paterson JC et al Serum lipid levels and the severity
of coronary and cerebral atherosclerosis in
adequately-nourished men, 60-69 years of age.
Medical Services Journal Canada. 1963 Jun; 19 : 410-20

Dr JC Paterson of the Westminster Hospital, London, Canada measured the cholesterol levels of 42 war veterans aged 60-69 over a 10 year period and again at post-mortem to investigate the relationship between cholesterol levels and blockage of the arteries.

This study found:

- There was NO correlation between cholesterol levels and the amount of blockage in the arteries.
- Those who had lower cholesterol had suffered from more previous heart attacks and blood clots than had those who had higher cholesterol.
- One man had a cholesterol level of only 111mg/dL (2.8 mmol/l). He had suffered a heart attack and had severe blockage of the arteries.

This study shows that the cholesterol/heart disease hypothesis is false.

Paper 7
Analysis of 1,700 patients finds NO association between the level of cholesterol in the blood and the incidence of heart disease

H. Edward Garrett, MD; Evan C. Horning, PhD; Billy G. Creech, PhD; Michael De-Bakey, MD Serum Cholesterol Values in Patients Treated Surgically for Atherosclerosis. *Journal of the American Medical Association.* 1964; 189(9) : 655-659

Michael Elias DeBakey (September 7, 1908 – July 11, 2008) was a world-renowned Lebanese-American cardiac surgeon, innovator, scientist, medical educator, and international medical statesman. DeBakey was the chancellor emeritus of Baylor College of Medicine in Houston, Texas and director of The Methodist DeBakey Heart & Vascular Centre and senior attending surgeon of The Methodist Hospital in Houston.

This analysis of the cholesterol values of 1,700 patients with heart disease conducted by Michael DeBakey, found NO association between the level of cholesterol in the blood and the incidence of heart disease.

Paper 8
Another study finds that cholesterol levels are NOT connected to clogged arteries

Jose Mendez et al Relationship between Serum Lipids and Aortic Atherosclerotic Lesions in Sudden Accidental Deaths in Guatemala City. *American Journal of Clinical Nutrition.* Vol 20, 1113-1117

Post-mortem blood samples were collected from 43 individuals, who died suddenly in accidents in Guatemala City, within two to 5 hours after death from the Institute of Nutrition of Central America and Panama, Guatemala.

These samples revealed there was no connection between cholesterol levels at death and clogged arteries.

The papers in this chapter demonstrate how the diet/cholesterol/heart hypothesis is firstly; based on flawed and biased studies, and secondly; has been proved to be simply not true by Lande's study in 1936 and a raft of investigations in the 1960s that clearly show that blood cholesterol levels have no association with blockages in the arteries.

O.K. you might exclaim, but what about dietary cholesterol and fat, especially saturated fat, surely eating that must lead to an increased risk of heart disease? I mean isn't that what we are told on the radio and TV, and in the newspapers all the time?

The next chapter answers the questions about the relationship between dietary fat and cholesterol and heart disease.

CHAPTER 2

Dietary cholesterol and saturated fat lower the rates of heart disease

Doctors and health care workers have religiously preached the *avoid saturated fat; eat low fat dogma* now for decades. However where has it got us? Childhood obesity has more than tripled since 1976 and adult obesity rates have doubled. The amount of people with diabetes has gone through the roof, heart disease incidence has risen, and diseases such as asthma, ADHD, Alzheimer's and Parkinson's, which were once rare are now commonplace.

This chapter examines the role that dietary fat and cholesterol play in heart disease. If you take note of what emanates through the media you will do your best to avoid food high in fat and cholesterol.

However, is what you hear in the media correct?

What does the scientific literature say?

Let's take a look.

Paper 9
An increase in dietary fat and cholesterol is associated with less heart disease

Oglesby P et al A Longitudinal Study
of Coronary Heart Disease. *Circulation.*
1963; 28 : 20-31

1,989 men (initially free from heart disease) from the Hawthorne Works of the Western Electric Company were analysed for four years at the University of Illinois College of Medicine to record the incidence of heart disease. Fat and cholesterol intake was compared between the men who developed heart disease and the men who remained free from heart disease. In the study 88 men developed heart disease.

The study revealed:

- The average daily intake of saturated fat was identical in both the men who developed heart disease and the men who were free from heart disease.
- The men who developed heart disease consumed slightly less daily total animal fats than the men who were free from heart disease.
- The men who developed heart disease consumed less daily cholesterol than the men who were free from heart disease.

The study pinpointed that an increase in fat and dietary cholesterol was associated with less heart disease.

Paper 10
As saturated fat and cholesterol increase in the diet, then rates of heart attack and death decrease

Frantz ID et al Test of effect of lipid lowering by diet on cardiovascular risk. The Minnesota Coronary Survey. *Arteriosclerosis.* 1989 Jan-Feb; 9(1) : 129-35

The Minnesota Coronary Survey lasted for 4.5 years and compared the effects of two diets, cholesterol levels and the incidence of heart attacks, sudden deaths, and total deaths. The trial included 9,057 men and women.

The diets were either:

- ○ 39% fat control diet (18% saturated fat, 5% polyunsaturated fat, 16% monounsaturated fat, 446 mg dietary cholesterol per day) (High saturated fat, high cholesterol diet)
- ○ 38% fat treatment diet (9% saturated fat, 15% polyunsaturated fat, 14% monounsaturated fat, 166 mg dietary cholesterol per day) (Low saturated fat, low cholesterol diet)

Dr Frantz found:

- • Cholesterol levels remained similar on the high saturated fat, high cholesterol diet.
- • Cholesterol levels fell by 16% on the low saturated fat, low cholesterol diet.
- • Those on the low saturated fat, low cholesterol diet had a 5% increased risk of a heart attack and sudden

death compared to those on the high saturated fat, high cholesterol diet.

• Those on the low saturated fat, low cholesterol diet had a 6% increase in death rates compared to those on the high saturated fat, high cholesterol diet.

This study reveals that as animal fat and animal protein increase in the diet, then rates of heart attack and death decrease.

Paper 11
Dietary cholesterol does NOT increase the risk of developing clogged arteries in pre-menopausal women

Herron KL et al Pre-menopausal women, classified as hypo- or hyper-responders, do not alter their LDL/HDL ratio following a high dietary cholesterol challenge. *Journal of the American College of Nutrition.* 2002 Jun; 21(3) : 250-8

In this study based at the Department of Nutritional Sciences, University of Connecticut, 51 pre-menopausal women aged 18 to 49 were given either 640 mg additional dietary cholesterol per day (by eggs) or a placebo group who had no additional dietary cholesterol, for 30 days to evaluate the effect of cholesterol on the arteries.

In some women the extra dietary cholesterol had no effect on their cholesterol levels, whereas in others there was a rise. However in the others, the eggs produced a rise in the "good" high-density lipoprotein (HDL) cholesterol which gives protection from heart disease (*see papers 54, 55, 56, 57, 58, 59*).

Herron concluded that excess dietary cholesterol does not increase the risk of developing clogged arteries in pre-menopausal women.

Paper 12
Diets high in cholesterol and saturated fat lower the risk of heart disease and diabetes

Bermudez O et al Dietary and plasma lipid, lipoprotein, and apolipoprotein profiles among elderly Hispanics and non-Hispanics and their association with diabetes. *American Journal of Clinical Nutrition.* 2002 Dec; 76(6) : 1214-21

The objective of the study was to assess the dietary and cholesterol risk factors for cardiovascular disease and their relationship to diabetes. The study involved 490 Hispanics and 163 non-Hispanic whites aged 60-98 years. The study was headed by Dr Odilia Bermudez who is an Assistant Professor at Tufts University.

After studying the dietary data Dr Bermudez found that:

- Hispanics ate more carbohydrate and polyunsaturated fats than non-Hispanic whites.
- Hispanics ate less cholesterol and saturated and monounsaturated fats than non-Hispanic whites.

Measurements of the heart protective high density lipoprotein (HDL) cholesterol *(see paper 54)* and heart protective apolipoprotein A-1 *(see paper 56)* were analysed and the results showed that:

- The Hispanic subjects; who ate more carbohydrate and polyunsaturated fats and less cholesterol and saturated and monounsaturated fats, had lower levels of the heart protective high-density lipoprotein (HDL) cholesterol and heart protective apolipoprotein A-1.

* High levels of (bad) triglycerides *(see paper 88)* and low levels of (good) HDL cholesterol were more prevalent among Hispanics with diabetes than without diabetes.

The study results indicate that a diet high in cholesterol, saturated and monounsaturated fat, and low in carbohydrate and polyunsaturated fat lower the risk of heart disease and diabetes.

Paper 13
High cholesterol diet results in LESS
heart disease risk for men and women

Herron KL et al High intake of cholesterol results in less atherogenic low-density lipoprotein particles in men and women independent of response classification. Metabolism. 2004 Jun; 53(6) : 823-30

A second study was conducted by Kristin Herron from the University of Connecticut to investigate the effects of cholesterol on heart disease. In this trial 52 subjects, 27 women and 25 men (18 to 50 years) had again either 640 mg/d additional dietary cholesterol (by eggs) or no additional dietary cholesterol diet for 30 days.

Herron discovered that the subjects on the additional cholesterol diet produced less of the (bad) type B low-density lipoprotein (LDL) cholesterol *(see paper 91)* and more of the relatively benign type A LDL cholesterol.

Therefore this study reveals that higher amounts of dietary cholesterol may lower the risk of heart disease.

Paper 14
Vegetarians have a higher risk of heart disease compared to meat eaters

Kwok T et al Vascular Dysfunction in Chinese
Vegetarians: An Apparent Paradox?
Journal of the American College
of Cardiology. 2005; 46 : 1957-1958

Professor Timothy Kwok and his team from the Prince of Wales Hospital, Hong Kong investigated the following heart disease risk factors in 49 vegetarians and 49 omnivores (meat eaters):

- Carotid intima-media thickness (a measurement of the combined thicknesses of the intimal and medial layers of the carotid artery walls-so the greater the carotid intima-media thickness, the greater the risk of heart disease).
- Flow-mediated dilation of brachial artery (a measurement of blood flow in the brachial artery-the less the flow the greater the risk of heart disease).
- Vitamin B12 levels (low levels are associated with increased heart disease risk).
- Homocysteine levels (high levels are associated with increased heart disease risk) *(see paper 79)*.
- Blood pressure (high levels are associated with increased heart disease risk).

The dietary composition was compared and it was revealed that the vegetarians ate significantly less saturated fat, cholesterol and protein compared to the omnivores

The study identified:

- Vegetarians had significantly greater carotid intima-media thickness than omnivores.
- Vegetarians had less flow-mediated dilation of the brachial artery than omnivores.
- Vegetarians had lower vitamin B12 levels than omnivores.
- Vegetarians had higher homocysteine levels than omnivores.
- Vegetarians had higher blood pressure than omnivores.

In all five heart disease risk factors vegetarians had a higher risk of heart disease.

The study ascertained that vegetarians ate significantly less saturated fat, cholesterol and protein compared to the meat eaters, and that vegetarians have higher a risk of heart disease, so it follows that a diet low in saturated fat, cholesterol and protein will lead to higher rates of heart disease.

Conversely you could deduce; a diet high in saturated fat, cholesterol and protein will give protection from heart disease.

Paper 15
Dietary cholesterol in eggs gives multiple health benefits

Fernandez, ML Dietary cholesterol provided by eggs and plasma lipoproteins in healthy populations. Current Opinion in Clinical Nutrition & Metabolic Care. January 2006 Volume 9 Issue 1 p 8-12

Professor Fernandez holds a position in the Department of Nutritional Sciences at the University of Connecticut and has been an associate editor of the *Journal of Nutrition* since 2001.

In this paper she reviews the literature to examine if there is an association between egg consumption and heart disease.

Her findings were:

- Extensive research has not established a link between egg consumption and risk for coronary heart disease.
- Egg intake has been shown to promote the formation of the large relatively benign type A low-density lipoprotein (LDL) cholesterol, rather than the dangerous type B LDL cholesterol *(see paper 91)*.
- Eggs are also good sources of antioxidants known to protect the eye.

Professor Fernandez concludes: "We need to acknowledge that diverse healthy populations experience no risk in developing coronary heart disease by increasing their intake of cholesterol but, in contrast, they may have multiple beneficial effects by the inclusion of eggs in their regular diet".

Paper 16
A review of recent scientific data clearly demonstrates that dietary cholesterol is NOT correlated with increased risk for heart disease

Fernandez ML Rethinking dietary cholesterol. *Current Opinion in Clinical Nutrition and Metabolic Care.* 2011 Oct 26

5 years after her review on eggs and cholesterol Professor Maria Fernandez reviewed the recent evidence that challenges the current (low) recommended dietary restrictions regarding cholesterol consumption.

The review found:

- The data clearly demonstrates that dietary cholesterol is not correlated with increased risk for heart disease.
- In 75% of the population excessive cholesterol consumption does not raise the levels of blood cholesterol.
- In the other 25% of the population excessive cholesterol consumption does raise blood cholesterol levels, however it raises levels of (the good) high-density lipoprotein (HDL) cholesterol, so there is no increase in risk of heart disease.

Professor Fernandez states that the current recommendations limiting dietary cholesterol should be reconsidered.

Paper 17
Dietary fat is not responsible for heart disease

Mann GV Cardiovascular disease in the Masai.
Journal of Atherosclerosis Research.
Volume 4, Issue 4, 8 July 1964, Pages 289-312

Dr George Mann, now retired, was previously a professor in medicine and biochemistry at Vanderbilt University in Tennessee.

Dr Mann investigated the relationship between diet and heart disease in 400 Masai men and additional women and children.

His research uncovered:

- Masai men had a diet of exclusively meat and milk.
- They had NO heart disease.

Dr Mann concluded that dietary fat couldn't possibly be responsible for heart disease.

Paper 18
Restriction of saturated fat leads
to higher rates of heart disease
Rose GA Corn Oil for Ischaemic Heart Disease.
British Medical Journal. 12 June 1965 p. 1507

80 patients with heart disease were allocated at random to one of three diets by Dr Rose as a treatment for heart attacks and angina. After two years data was collected to find how many were still living and free from any fresh heart disease.

The three diets were:

- Group I continued their usual diet. They continued to eat as much animal fat, milk, butter and eggs as they desired *(High animal fat diet).*
- Groups II were instructed to avoid foods rich in animal fat and to restrict their intake of milk, butter, and eggs and received a daily supplement of 80 g of olive oil, which is rich in the monounsaturated oleic acid *(Olive oil and restriction of animal fat diet).*
- Groups III were instructed to avoid foods rich in animal fat and to restrict their intake of milk, butter, and eggs and received a similar quantity of corn oil,

which is rich in the polyunsaturated linoleic acid *(Corn oil and restriction of animal fat diet).*

The study found:

- Cholesterol levels remained steady in the high animal fat diet and olive oil diet.
- Cholesterol levels fell by 20-30 mg per 100 ml in the corn oil diet.
- More people were still living and free of any fresh heart disease in the high animal fat diet.
- More people died and suffered from fresh heart disease on the corn oil diet.
- After two years the proportion of patients alive and free of fresh heart disease was:
  Group 1. 75% *(high animal fat diet).*
  Group 2. 57% *(olive oil diet and restriction of fat & dairy).*
  Group 3. 52% *(corn oil diet and restriction of fat & dairy).*

At the end of the trial more people were still living and free of any fresh heart disease in the high animal fat diet compared to the olive oil and corn oil diet.

The results of this study show that restriction of saturated fat in the diet leads to higher rates of heart disease.

In other words, saturated fat offers protection from heart disease.

Paper 19
High saturated fat diets are associated with virtually NO heart disease

Prior IA et al Cholesterol, coconuts, and diet on Polynesian atolls: a natural experiment: the Pukapuka and Tokelau island studies. *American Journal of Clinical Nutrition.* Vol 34, 1552-1561

Dr Ian Prior, cardiologist and director of the epidemiology unit at Wellington Hospital in New Zealand, and his colleagues investigated the effects of saturated fat in determining cholesterol levels and heart disease in twopopulations of Polynesians (Pukapuka and Tokelau) living on atolls near the equator.

The research established:

- ○ The diets in both Pukapuka and Tokelau are high in saturated fat.
- ○ Tokelauans obtain a much higher percentage of energy from coconut than the Pukapukans, 63% compared with 34%, so their intake of saturated fat is higher.
- ○ The cholesterol levels are 35 to 40 mg higher in Tokelauans than in Pukapukans.
- ○ Heart disease was virtually non-existent in both groups.
- ○ The migration of Tokelau Islanders to New Zealand was associated with an increased risk for heart disease. After migration their diets changed-They ate less saturated fat and more carbohydrate.

If we examine the findings of the study we see:

- Dr Prior found that both groups ate diets high in saturated fats-*and had no heart disease.*
- Tokelauans ate more saturated fat, had higher cholesterol-*and had no heart disease.*
- After migrating to New Zealand, Tokelauans ate less saturated fat and more carbohydrate-*and suffered from heart disease.*

This study shows that high levels of saturated fat in the diet are associated with virtually no heart disease and when people lower their dietary saturated fat they suffer from heart disease.

Paper 20
Saturated fat consumption improves beneficial HDL cholesterol levels

Newbold HL Reducing the serum cholesterol level with a diet high in animal fat. *Southern Medical Journal.* 1988 Jan; 81(1) : 61-3

Multiple food allergies required a group of seven patients to follow a diet in which most of the calories came from beef fat. Their diets contained no sucrose, milk, or grains.

Dr Newbold measured several heart disease risk factors over the course of the study.

An analysis of his findings included:

- The patients' (bad) triglyceride *(see paper 88)* levels decreased from an average of 113 mg/dl to an average of 74 mg/dl.
- At the beginning of the study, six of the patients had an average (of the beneficial) high-density lipoprotein cholesterol (HDL) percentage of 21%. At the end of the study, the average had risen to 32%.

The study found that beneficial HDL cholesterol levels were improved on a high saturated fat diet. High HDL cholesterol levels can protect against heart disease *(see paper 57).*

These beneficial effects of saturated fat were confirmed in a study conducted by Dr Malcolm Kendrick (a general practitioner from Scotland).

He analyzed World Health Organisation data to find the saturated fat consumption and heart disease rates throughout the countries of Europe. He then grouped them into the seven countries with the lowest consumption of saturated fat, and compared this to their rate of heart disease, and also grouped the seven countries with the highest consumption of saturated fat and compared this to their rate of heart disease

His first seven countries were those with the lowest consumption of saturated fat. These were Georgia, Tajikistan, Azerbaijan, Moldova, Croatia, Macedonia and the Ukraine.

Kendrick's second seven countries were those with the highest consumption of saturated fat. These were Austria, Finland, Belgium, Iceland, Netherlands, Switzerland and France.

Every single one of the seven countries with the *lowest* consumption of saturated fat had significantly *higher* heart disease than every single one of the countries with the *highest* consumption of saturated fat.

Paper 21
Analysis of 27 trials finds the best way to raise HDL (good cholesterol) is to eat saturated fat

Mensink RP Effect of dietary fatty acids on serum lipids and lipoproteins. A meta-analysis of 27 trials
Arteriosclerosis and Thrombosis. Vol 12, 911-919

Ronald P Mensink is a Professor of Molecular Nutrition with emphasis on lipid metabolism at the Maastricht University Medical Centre.

Professor Mensink reviewed 27 studies to calculate the effect of replacing carbohydrates with either saturated fat, monounsaturated fat or polyunsaturated fat on (the beneficial) high-density lipoprotein (HDL) cholesterol levels and (the harmful) triglyceride levels.

Mensink's review discovered:

- All fats lowered the harmful triglyceride levels *(see paper 88)*.
- All fats raised the beneficial HDL cholesterol levels, but saturated fat raised it the most!

This review supports the concept that the best way to raise the heart protective HDL (good cholesterol) is to eat saturated fat, it therefore follows that a diet high in saturated fat is heart protective.

Paper 22
Increased saturated fat consumption leads to lower rates of heart disease and stroke

Serra-Majem L et al How could changes in diet explain changes in coronary heart disease mortality in Spain? The Spanish paradox. *American Journal of Clinical Nutrition.* Vol 61, 1351S-1359S

Professor Serra-Majem and his team from the University of Barcelona reviewed and compared trends in coronary heart disease and stroke mortality in Spain from 1966 to 1990 and changes in food consumption.

The review found that in Spain from 1966 to 1990:

- Rates of heart disease deaths fell.
- Rates of stroke death fell.
- There was an increase in meat consumption.
- There was a decrease in carbohydrate consumption.
- Fat and saturated fat intakes increased.

This review shows that an increase in consumption of saturated fat and meat, together with a decrease in consumption of carbohydrate led to lower rates of heart disease and stroke.

Paper 23
Men who eat the most saturated fat have a 27% DECREASE in heart disease deaths

Pietinen P et al Intake of Fatty Acids and Risk of Coronary Heart Disease in a Cohort of Finnish Men: The Alpha-Tocopherol, Beta-Carotene Cancer Prevention Study. *American Journal of Epidemiology.* (1997) 145 (10): 876-887

This study of six years, which was based at the Department of Nutrition, National Public Health Institute, Helsinki, Finland and headed by Professor Pirjo Pietinen, investigated the relationship between intakes of various fats and the risk of coronary heart disease in 21,930 smoking men aged 50–69 years who were initially free of diagnosed cardiovascular disease.

The study revealed:

- Those men who consumed the most polyunsaturated fats (vegetable oils, margarine etc) had a 27% increase in coronary death and an 11% increase in major coronary events compared to those men that consumed the least.

- Those men who consumed the most saturated fats had a 27% decrease in coronary death and a 13% decrease in major coronary events compared to those men that consumed the least.
- Those men who consumed the most cholesterol had a 8% decrease in coronary death and an 7% decrease in major coronary events compared to those men that consumed the least.

The results of this study indicate that polyunsaturated fats increase heart disease and that cholesterol and especially saturated fat consumption lower the incidence of heart disease.

Paper 24
Saturated fat lowers (bad)
Lp(a) cholesterol levels

Clevidence BA Plasma Lipoprotein (a) Levels in Men and Women Consuming Diets Enriched in Saturated, Cis-, or Trans-Monounsaturated Fatty Acids. *Arteriosclerosis, Thrombosis, and Vascular Biology.* 1997; 17 : 1657-1661

High lipoprotein (a) [Lp(a)] cholesterol levels are associated with heart disease *(see papers 84 and 85).*

Dr Clevidence officiated over this study which set out to determine the effect on Lp(a) levels by four different diets. The trial included 29 men and 29 women and lasted for 6 weeks.

The diets consisted of:

- A high monounsaturated diet.
- A moderate trans fat diet.
- A high trans fat diet.
- A high saturated fat diet.

The study revealed that the saturated fat diet lowered dangerous Lp(a) levels *(see paper 85)* significantly(by 8% to 11%) and therefore reduced heart disease risk.

Paper 25
Increasing dietary saturated fat
may help you to live longer

Ravnskov U The Questionable Role of Saturated and
Polyunsaturated Fatty Acids in Cardiovascular Disease.
Journal of Clinical Epidemiology. Volume 51,
Issue 6, June 1998, Pages 443-460

Dr Ravnskov is a scientist and has published more than 80 papers and letters in the scientific press critical to the cholesterol campaign, for which he has won two international awards.

Ravnskov reviewed the evidence concerning the hypothesis that a fat diet, rich in saturated fat and low in polyunsaturated fat, is said to be an important cause of atherosclerosis and cardiovascular diseases.

His review revealed:

- In larger studies, there tended to be no correlation between saturated fat intake and cardiovascular mortality and even a trend towards lower death rates.

- Trends of national fat consumption and death from coronary heart disease in 18–35 countries (four studies) during different time periods diverged from each other as often as they coincided.
- In 14 other studies:
- 1 study supported the hypothesis.
- 6 studies gave partly supportive, partly contradictive results.
- 7 studies did not support the hypothesis.
- In a meta-analysis of nine controlled randomised dietary trials with substantial reductions of dietary fats, neither heart disease or total death rates were lowered.

The evidence from Dr Ravnskov's review almost completely rejected the hypothesis that a fat diet, rich in saturated fat and low in polyunsaturated fat, is said to be an important cause of atherosclerosis and cardiovascular diseases.

The review rather more tended to support the hypothesis that saturated fat may offer a protective effect from heart disease.

Ravnskov concluded, rather understatedly: *"The harmful effect of dietary saturated fat and the protective effect of dietary polyunsaturated fat on atherosclerosis and heart disease are questioned"*.

Paper 26
High animal protein intake associated with a lower risk of heart disease for women

Hu FB et al Dietary protein and risk of ischemic heart disease in women. *American Journal of Clinical Nutrition.* Vol. 70, No. 2, 221-227, August 1999

The objective of this Harvard study was to examine the relationship between protein intake and risk of ischemic heart disease. The trial included 80,082 women aged 34–59 and lasted for 14 years.

The study found that those with the highest protein intake had a 26% decreased risk of ischemic heart disease compared to those with the lowest intake and animal protein (accompanied by increases in saturated fat and cholesterol intake) contributed towards this decreased risk.

Paper 27
Saturated fat helps to reduce
heart disease risk factors

Kratz M et al Dietary Mono- and Polyunsaturated Fatty Acids Similarly Affect LDL Size in Healthy Men and Women. *Journal of Nutrition.* 132:715-718, 2002

The goal of this German study was to investigate the effects of dietary monounsaturated, polyunsaturated and saturated Fats on low-density lipoprotein (LDL) cholesterol size. The study included 56 (30 men, 26 women) healthy participants.

First, all participants received a diet rich in saturated fat for two weeks and LDL size was measured; they were then randomly assigned to one of three oil dietary treatments for four weeks and again LDL size was measured.

The three diets on the oil phase were either:

- Olive oil rich in monounsaturated fat.
- Rapeseed oil rich in monounsaturated fat and polyunsaturated fat.
- Sunflower oil rich in polyunsaturated fat.

Analysis revealed a significant reduction in LDL size during the four week oil diet phase.

Kratz concluded that all dietary unsaturated fat reduced LDL size compared to saturated fat.

Compared with small LDL cholesterol, having more large size LDL cholesterol gives protection from heart disease and diabetes *(see paper 91).*

The results of the study portray how saturated fat may again give protection from heart disease.

Paper 28
High fat diet reduces heart disease risk and helps in weight loss

Foster GD et al A Randomized Trial of a Low-Carbohydrate Diet for Obesity. *New England Journal of Medicine.* Volume 348:2082-2090 May 22, 2003 Number 21

In this study published in the *New England Journal of Medicine* Professor Gary Foster conducted a one-year trial on 63 obese men and women to ascertain the effects of two different diets on triglycerides, weight loss and the levels of the heart friendly high-density lipoprotein (HDL) cholesterol *(see papers 54-59).*

The diets were either:

- Low-carbohydrate, high-protein, high-fat diet.
- Low-calorie, high-carbohydrate, low-fat diet.

The study found:

- Those on the high fat diet lost more weight than those on the low fat diet.
- Those on the high fat diet had a bigger increase in the beneficial HDL cholesterol compared to those on the low fat diet.
- Those on the high fat diet had a bigger decrease in dangerous triglyceride levels *(see paper 88)* compared to those on the low fat diet.

Professor Foster concluded that the high fat diet produced a greater weight loss and was associated with a greater improvement in HDL cholesterol and triglyceride levels and therefore lowered the risk of heart disease.

Paper 29
Patients enjoy improved cholesterol and weight loss on a high saturated fat diet

Hays JH Effect of a High Saturated Fat and No-Starch Diet on Serum Lipid Sub-fractions in Patients With Documented Atherosclerotic Cardiovascular Disease.
Mayo Clinic Proceedings. 2003; 78 : 1331-1336

Cardiology researchers from Newark enrolled 23 obese non-diabetic patients with cardiovascular disease on a six-week trial to determine the effects of a high saturated fat and avoidance of starch diet (HSF-SA), on weight loss and cholesterol levels.

Also 15 obese patients with polycystic ovary syndrome and eight obese patients with reactive hypoglycaemia were monitored during an HSF-SA diet for 24 and 52 weeks, respectively.

The study found:

- Patients with cardiovascular disease lost 5.2% of their bodyweight.
- Dangerous triglyceride levels decreased *(see paper 88)*.
- Dangerous very low-density lipoprotein (VLDL) levels decreased *(see paper 90)*.
- Low-density level lipoproteins (LDL) changed from (the bad) small and dense type to the more healthy large and fluffy type *(see paper 91)*.
- Patients with polycystic ovary syndrome lost 14.3% of their bodyweight and patients with reactive hypoglycaemia lost 19.9% of their bodyweight at 24 and 52 weeks, respectively, without any adverse effects on their lipoprotein levels.

The high saturated fat diet improved the cholesterol profile of the patients, and they also experienced a substantial weight loss, hence they lowered their risk of heart disease.

Paper 30
Saturated fat lowers the risk of heart disease

Volek JS et al The case for not restricting saturated fat on a low carbohydrate diet. *Nutrition & Metabolism.* 2005; 2 : 21

Jeff Volek is a dietician-scientist and an associate professor at the University of Connecticut. He has also contributed to over 200 scientific papers.

In this paper Volek examined the effects of saturated fat on heart disease risk markers.

He found:

- Saturated fat does not raise (bad) LDL cholesterol levels.
- Saturated fat actually slowed down the progression of "clogged arteries".
- Saturated fat increases (good) HDL cholesterol, *(see papers 54-59)* decreases (bad) triglycerides *(see paper 88)* and increases the particle size of LDL cholesterol from a small dense dangerous type B, to a large fluffy relatively benign type A *(see paper 91)*.
- When saturated fat is replaced by carbohydrates undesirable effects occur such as an increase in (bad) triglycerides with a decrease in (good) HDL cholesterol.

This paper demonstrates how saturated fat can lower the risk of heart disease.

Paper 31
Red meat gives protection from heart disease
Mamo JC et al A low-protein diet exacerbates postprandial chylomicron concentration in moderately dyslipidaemic subjects in comparison to a lean red meat protein-enriched diet. *European Journal of Clinical Nutrition* 2005 Oct: 59(10) : 1142-8

Professor John Mamo, a professor of health sciences at Curtin University, Australia and his colleagues investigated the implications on heart disease risk of diets either low in protein (14, 53 and 30% of energy as protein, carbohydrate and fat, respectively) or high in protein (red meat) (25, 35 and 30% energy as protein, carbohydrate and fat) in 20 people for a period of six weeks.

The study revealed that those on the low protein diet had increased (bad) chylomicrons in the bloodstream. Mamo concluded that the red meat helped to curtail the excess chylomicrons.

Elevated chylomicrons are associated with heart disease *(see paper 86)*.

Paper 32
High saturated fat diets
DECREASE heart disease risk factors

Noakes M et al Comparison of isocaloric very low carbohydrate/high saturated fat and high carbohydrate/low saturated fat diets on body composition and cardiovascular risk. *Nutrition and Metabolism.* 2006; 3 : 7

The objective of this study, headed by Dr Manny Noakes a senior research scientist at the Commonwealth Scientific and Industrial Research Organisation, was to compare, the effects of a high saturated fat very low carbohydrate diet against two low saturated fat high carbohydrate diets, on body composition and cardiovascular risk in 83 subjects average age 48 years.

The diets composed of:

- ○ High saturated fat/very low carbohydrate diet: (4% carbohydrate, 35% protein, 61% fat, of which 20% was saturated).
- ○ High unsaturated fat diet: (50% carbohydrate, 20% protein, 30% fat, of which 6% was saturated).
- ○ Very low fat diet: (70% carbohydrate, 20% protein, 10% fat, of which 3% was saturated).

Dr Noakes found:

- Subjects lost more weight on the high saturated fat/very low carbohydrate diet compared to the other two diets.
- (The good) High Density Lipoprotein (HDL) Cholesterol *(see papers 54-59)* increased on the high saturated fat/very low carbohydrate diet, relative to the other two diets.
- (The bad) triglycerides *(see paper 88)* were lowered on the high saturated fat/very low carbohydrate diet, but actually increased on the other two diets.
- The high saturated fat/very low carbohydrate diet lowered (the bad) fasting insulin levels *(see paper 78)* by 33%. The high unsaturated fat diet lowered fasting insulin by 19% and the very low fat diet had no effect.
- The high saturated fat/very low carbohydrate diet also provoked significantly lower post meal glucose and insulin responses than the very low fat and high unsaturated fat meals.

The study shows that high saturated fat/very low carbohydrate diets decrease heart disease risk factors.

Paper 33
Almost all epidemiological and experimental studies show that a reduction in saturated fat has NO health benefits

Ravnskov U Is saturated fat bad?
Nutrition and Health. 2010; Part 2, 109-119

Dr Uffe Ranvskov is known as the expert's expert on the subject of saturated fat, cholesterol and heart disease.

In this paper Dr Ravnskov notes that for decades a reduction of the intake of saturated fat has been the cornerstone in dietary prevention of cardiovascular disease. The main argument for this advice is its alleged influence on blood cholesterol.

However in this review Ravnskov found:

- Several recent trials have found that saturated fat intake has no such effect on cholesterol in spite of fat intakes of up to five times higher than the recommended upper limit.
- Ravnskov assessed the assumption "a high intake of saturated fat is harmful and a reduction leads to health benefits". He found: Almost all epidemiological and experimental studies are in conflict with this assumption; indeed several observations points to the opposite.

As evidence points to the fact that a higher saturated fat intake may lead to health benefits, Dr Ravnskov concludes there is an urgent need for a revision of the present dietary guidelines which advise a very low limit of saturated fat consumption.

Paper 34
Analysis of 347,747 people finds that eating saturated fat has NO association with heart disease

Siri-Tarino et al Meta-analysis of prospective cohort studies evaluating the association of saturated fat with cardiovascular disease. *American Journal of Clinical Nutrition.*
January 13, 2010 Mar; 91(3) : 535-46

A research team headed by Patty Siri-Tarino examined the scientific literature on the subject of saturated fat and heart disease.

They found 21 studies, which had lasted between 5-23 years and included 347,747 people.

After analysing all this data they found that saturated fat consumption had NO association with heart disease.

Paper 35
Lard offers protection from heart disease compared to olive oil

Teng KT et al Palm olein and olive oil cause a higher increase in postprandial Teng KT lipemia compared with lard but had no effect on plasma glucose, insulin and adipocytokines.
Lipids. 2011 Apr; 46(4) : 381-8

High triglyceride levels measured after meals have the strongest association with heart attacks and cardiovascular events *(see paper 88).*

This study of 10 healthy men was designed to compare the effects of 50g of fat on triglyceride levels from either:

○ Palm olein.
○ Lard.
○ Virgin olive oil.
○ The study found that triglyceride concentrations were significantly lower after the lard meal than after the olive oil and palm olein meals.

The study findings reveal that lard offers protection from heart disease compared to olive oil and palm olein.

Further confirmation of the findings that lard is heart protective, is the fact that lard is the second richest dietary source of vitamin D and that low levels of vitamin D have been linked to an increased heart disease risk.

Paper 36
High saturated fat diet can lower
the risk of heart attack and stroke

Wood AC et al Dietary Carbohydrate Modifies
the Inverse Association Between Saturated Fat
Intake and Cholesterol on Very Low-Density Lipoproteins.
Lipid Insights. 2011 August 23; 2011(4) : 7–15

Having high triglyceride and high Very Low Density Lipoprotein (VLDL) cholesterol levels means you may have an increased risk of coronary artery disease, which can lead to a heart attack or stroke *(see papers 88, 90)*.

This study at the University of Alabama investigated the relationship between dietary saturated fat, and triglyceride and Very Low Density Lipoprotein cholesterol levels in 1036 men and women, average age 49.

- The study found that: The higher the saturated fat intake in the diet, the lower the triglyceride and Very Low Density Lipoprotein cholesterol levels when subjects consumed a low carbohydrate diet. This was not the case at higher intakes of carbohydrate.

The study shows that a high saturated fat diet can decrease risk factors pertaining to heart attack and stroke when consumed with a low carbohydrate diet.

Paper 37
A high saturated fat diet increases
the levels of the beneficial HDL cholesterol
Siri-Tarino PW Effects of Diet on High-Density Lipoprotein Cholesterol. *Current Atherosclerosis Reports* 2011 Dec; 13(6) :453-60

The American Heart Association give the advice that high-density lipoprotein cholesterol (HDL-C) is the "good cholesterol" and may help to prevent heart disease.

In this paper Siri-Tarino reviewed the effects of various diets on HDL-C levels.

Siri-Tarino found:

- Added sugars were associated with decreased HDL-C levels.
- HDL-C levels were increased by 4-5% with weight loss, omega-3 fatty acids, and a Mediterranean diet pattern.

- Replacement of dietary carbohydrate with polyunsaturated fats is associated with a 7% increase in HDL-C.
- Replacement of dietary carbohydrate with saturated fats is associated with a 12% increase in HDL-C. (Monosaturated fats effects were in-between the polyunsaturated and saturated values).

This study proves again that the best way to raise the levels of beneficial high-density lipoprotein (HDL) cholesterol is to eat a diet rich in saturated fat.

Paper 38
Meat helps to treat heart disease

Lerman A et al L-Arginine: a novel therapy for coronary artery disease? *Expert Opinion on Investigational Drugs.* 1999 Nov; 8(11) : 1785-1793

Dr Amir Lerman specialises in interventional cardiology in cardiovascular disease at the Mayo Clinic, Rochester.

Dr Lerman states that the endothelium (the thin layer of cells that lines the interior surface of blood vessels) needs to stay intact to function correctly. When the endothelium is compromised, endothelial dysfunction may occur which may be a precursor to heart disease.

L-Arginine is a semi-essential amino acid that improves endothelial function and can give protection from heart disease.

The best dietary sources of L-Arginine are beef, pork, gelatin, poultry, wild game, seafood and dairy products.

Paper 39
Compounds richly available in meat
can improve heart function

Allard ML et al The management of conditioned nutritional
requirements in heart failure. *Heart Failure Reviews.*
2006 Mar; 11(1) : 75-82

This review was carried out by researchers at the
University Health Network in Toronto.

The researchers demonstrated how patients suffering
from congestive heart failure have lowered heart energy
production, and higher cell and muscle damage.

Nutritional factors known to be important for these
conditions, such as thiamine, riboflavin, pyridoxine,
L-carnitine, coenzyme Q10, creatine and taurine are
deficient in patients with heart failure.

Meat is a rich source of thiamine, riboflavin, pyridoxine,
L-carnitine, coenzyme Q10, creatine and taurine.

Dietary consumption of these compounds in heart failure
can significantly restore depleted levels and may result in
improvement in heart structure and function as well as
exercise capacity.

Paper 40
Taurine may help prevent heart disease

Tan B et al Taurine protects against low-density lipoprotein-
induced endothelial dysfunction by the DDAH/ADMA
pathway. *Vascular Pharmacology.* 2007 May; 46(5) : 338-45

Here's another paper that describes the importance of the endothelium.

Tan explains that the endothelium is the thin layer of cells that lines the interior surface of blood vessels. Endothelial dysfunction is a process in which the endothelium secretes substances that promote an artery-clogging build-up of plaque rather than the protective substances that prevent this build-up. It is the earliest detectable stage of cardiovascular disease.

Tan and his team tested the effects of taurine on endothelial dysfunction.

They discovered that taurine has a protective effect.

This paper suggests that taurine may help to stop the arteries clogging up.

The best dietary sources of taurine are meat and fish.

This chapter has shown that far from increasing the rates of heart disease, saturated fat and dietary cholesterol help in reducing the rates of heart disease!

Countless papers report that a high consumpive of saturated fat and cholesterol leads to increases in the heart protective High Density Lipoprotein (HDL) cholesterol.

Invariably eating high amounts of saturated fat in the diet also lowers the levels of the heart damaging types of cholesterol (more on this in chapter 4), and dangerously high levels of insulin and homocysteine are also reduced.

Eminent doctors have reviewed the available literature and come to the conclusion that saturated fat and dietary cholesterol are NOT heart dangerous, but in fact may be heart healthy.

The data shows that diets high in saturated fat are the best solution for weight loss.

Dietary cholesterol and saturated fat also improve blood flow.

Eating red meat means you will get copious amounts of nutrients such as L-arginine, taurine and co-enzyme Q10 that are essential for a healthy heart.

But what about in the "real world". Does eating a diet high in cholesterol and saturated fat reduce heart disease?

Studies have presented data that shows that when saturated fat and cholesterol consumption go up, then rates of heart disease go down.

Populations from rural Africa and Polynesia who eat copious amounts of saturated fat have been found to have virtually no heart disease – unless they move to urban environments, where they invariably cut their consumption of saturated fat, and then start to suffer heart problems.

This is also true of mainland Europe. In over a quarter of a century in Spain the consumption of saturated fat rose and rates of heart disease fell. In a Europe wide study, every one of the seven countries that consumed the most saturated fat had lower rates of heart disease than every one of the seven countries that consumed the least saturated fat.

Papers comparing those who eat the most saturated fat show they enjoy up to a 27% decrease in heart disease rates compared to those who eat the least saturated fat.

The scientific evidence has portrayed to us that dietary cholesterol and saturated fat do not cause heart disease and may in fact be heart protective.

But what about blood cholesterol levels? Aren't we always told that if we have high cholesterol then we will die earlier, probably of heart disease?

The next chapter addresses that question.

Chapter 3

High cholesterol
levels help you live longer

Listening to the commentary (and adverts) in the media you could be forgiven for thinking that cholesterol is an evil substance that must under all circumstances be eliminated from your body.

It seems that almost everyone over the age of 50 is prescribed a statin drug when they visit their doctor to lower their "dangerously high" cholesterol levels. This trend of taking statins is increasing in younger and younger age groups, and some doctors are even saying statins should be put in the water supply!

However what is a "dangerously high" cholesterol level?

Should we all be on cholesterol lowering medication?

Should we be trying to lower our cholesterol in the first place?

Read the following scientific evidence, and then make up your own mind.

Paper 41
A direct association between falling cholesterol levels and mortality in men and women aged between 31 and 65 years old

Anderson KM et al Cholesterol and mortality. 30 years of follow-up from the Framingham study.

Journal of the American Medical Association.

1987 Apr 24; 257(16) : 2176-80

The Framingham Heart Study is a long-term, ongoing cardiovascular study on residents of the town of Framingham, Massachusetts. The study began in 1948 with 5,209 adult subjects from Framingham, and is now on its third generation of participants.

In one of the trials associated with the Framingham Heart Study, cholesterol levels were measured in 1959 men and 2415 women aged between 31 and 65 years who were free of cardiovascular disease and cancer over a four year period.

After examining the results the researchers found:

- There is a direct association between falling cholesterol levels over the first 14 years and an increase in total death rates over the following 18 years (11% increase per 1 mg/dL per year drop in cholesterol levels).
- There is a direct association between falling cholesterol levels over the first 14 years and an increase in cardiovascular death rates over the following 18 years (14% increase per 1 mg/dL per year drop in cholesterol levels).

The paper illustrates that if your cholesterol levels fall you have a greatly increased risk of dying-and an even greater risk of dying from cardiovascular disease, and the more your cholesterol levels fall the bigger the risk of premature death.

Paper 42
Men given "healthy living" advice and cholesterol lowering drugs are twice as likely to die

Miettinen TA et al Multifactorial Primary Prevention of Cardiovascular Diseases in Middle-aged Men.
Journal of the American Medical Association.
1985; 254(15) : 2097-2102

This study, published in the *Journal of the American Medical Association* examined the effects of preventative measures for men with a high risk of heart disease and stroke. 1,222 men at high risk were split into two groups.

Group (i) The intervention group (612 men).

Group (ii) The high risk control group (610 men).

Group (iii) A third group of men with a low risk of heart disease and stroke were also analysed (593 men).

The subjects in the intervention group (i) were treated with a range of measures:

- They met up with the investigators every four months for five years.
- They were repeatedly given oral and written dietary advice.
- They were advised to reduce the intake of calories, saturated fat, cholesterol, alcohol, and sugar and to increase that of polyunsaturated fats (mainly soft margarine), fish, chicken, veal, and vegetables.

- A program to increase physical activity was given to every participant, and anti-smoking advice was given individually to all smokers.
- Cholesterol levels, blood pressure, and body weight were measured at each visit.
- If their cholesterol levels were high they were treated with cholesterol lowering drugs.
- If their blood pressure was high they were treated with blood pressure lowering drugs.

No advice or treatment was given to the subjects in the high risk control group (ii) and the low risk control group (iii).

The results of the study revealed:

- There were twice as many deaths in the intervention group (i) compared to the high risk control group (ii).
- There were four times as many cardiac deaths in the intervention group (i) compared to the high risk control group (ii).
- There was an 11% increase in non-fatal cardiovascular events (heart attack, stroke) in the intervention group (i) compared to the high risk control group (ii).

This study revealed that men who were given medications to lower their cholesterol and blood pressure levels and advice such as to reduce their saturated fat and cholesterol intake were twice as likely to die as men who were not, and also four times more likely to have cardiac deaths.

Paper 43
Lowering cholesterol levels does
not prevent coronary heart disease

Ravnskov U Cholesterol lowering trials in coronary
heart disease: Frequency of citation and outcome.
British Medical Journal. 305 : 15 4 July 1992

The objective of this review by Dr Ravnskov was to see if the claim that lowering cholesterol values prevents coronary heart disease is true, or if it is based on citation of supportive trials only.

After searching the literature Ravnskov found 22 controlled cholesterol lowering trials that measured coronary heart disease or death, or both.

This investigation revealed that:

- Trials considered as supportive of the contention that lowering cholesterol values prevents coronary heart disease were cited almost six times more often than others.
- Trials considered as unsupportive of the contention that lowering cholesterol values prevents coronary heart disease were not cited after 1970, although their number almost equalled the number considered supportive.
- In the 22 controlled cholesterol lowering trials studied, total mortality and coronary heart disease mortality was not changed significantly either overall or in any sub-group.
- Cholesterol levels were not related to heart disease.
- There was a significant increase in non-medical deaths in the cholesterol lowering groups.

Ravnskov concluded that lowering cholesterol levels does not reduce mortality and is unlikely to prevent coronary heart disease. Claims of the opposite are based on preferential citation of supportive trials.

Paper 44
Cholesterol levels have no
influence on heart disease or mortality

Krumholz HM et al Lack of association between cholesterol and coronary heart disease mortality and morbidity and all-cause mortality in persons older than 70 years. *Journal of the American Medical Association.* 1994 Nov 2; 272(17) : 1335-40

Dr Harlan Krumholz is a Professor of Medicine and Epidemiology and Public Health at Yale University School of Medicine.

Dr Krumholz presided over this study, of which the objective was to determine whether elevated cholesterol levels are associated with total death rates and heart disease in people older than 70.

Over four years 997 subjects had their cholesterol levels measured and they were divided into two groups:

- Low cholesterol group (less than 5.20 mmol/L or 200 mg/dL).
- High cholesterol group (above or equal to 6.20 mmol/L or 240 mg/dL).

Dr Krumholz and his team of researchers found:

- Death rates were similar-although the death rates in those who had the higher cholesterol was 1% less compared to those with the lower cholesterol.
- Cholesterol levels had no influence on rates of heart disease.

This study found that high cholesterol values do not cause heart disease or mortality in persons over 70 years.

Paper 45
Low cholesterol is associated with marked increase in mortality in heart failure

Horwich TB et al Low serum total cholesterol is associated with marked increase in mortality in advanced heart failure. *Journal of Cardiac Failure.* 2002 Aug; 8(4) : 216-24

This study, published in the *Journal of Cardiac Failure* investigated the relationship between cholesterol levels and heart failure.

Cholesterol levels were measured in 1,134 patients with advanced heart failure.

The study revealed that those with the lowest cholesterol had over double the risk of dying from advanced heart failure compared to those with the highest cholesterol.

Paper 46
In patients with chronic heart failure, lower total cholesterol levels are associated with earlier death

Rauchhaus M et al The relationship between cholesterol and survival in patients with chronic heart failure.
Journal of the American College of Cardiology.
2003; 42 : 1933-1940

The objective of this UK study was to find the relationship between cholesterol levels and survival in patients with chronic heart failure. A total of 417 patients were involved in the study.

The results of the study revealed:

- Higher total cholesterol levels were a predictor of survival.
- The chance of survival increased 25% for each mmol/l (38 mg/dl) increment in total cholesterol.
- After one year those with cholesterol levels above 5.2 mmol/l (201 mg/dL) had a survival rate of 92%.
- After one year those with cholesterol levels below 5.2 mmol/l (201 mg/dL) had a survival rate of 75%.
- After three years those with cholesterol levels above 5.2 mmol/l (201 mg/dL) had a survival rate of 72%.
- After three years those with cholesterol levels below 5.2 mmol/l (201 mg/dL) had a survival rate of 50%.

The data from this UK study shows that in patients with chronic heart failure, lower total cholesterol levels are associated with earlier death.

Paper 47
Low cholesterol levels are strongly associated with increased mortality in patients with nonischemic, systolic heart failure

Afsarmanesh N et al Total cholesterol levels and mortality risk in nonischemic systolic heart failure. *American Heart Journal.* 2006 Dec; 152(6) : 1077-83

- Nonischemic heart disease is a disease of the heart that lacks the associated coronary artery disease often found in other diseases of the heart. It's usually linked to a disease in one or more of the cardiac muscles, causing the heart to pump in an ineffective manner, thereby reducing the transport of blood, oxygen and other nutrients throughout the body. One of the more common nonischemic heart diseases is dilated cardiomyopathy. In this form of heart disease, your left ventricle has weakened (low left ventricular ejection fraction (LVEF)) to the point where it can no longer pump enough blood.
- Hemodynamics is a measurement of blood pressure and blood flow.
- The New York Heart Association (NYHA) Functional Classification provides a simple way of classifying the extent of heart failure. It places patients in one of four classes based on how much they are limited during physical activity. E.g. Class one indicates: *No symptoms and no limitation in ordinary physical activity*, whilst class four is defined as: *Severe limitations. Experiences symptoms even while at rest. Mostly bedbound patients.*

The study analyzed the cholesterol levels of 614 patients with nonischemic systolic heart failure who had a left ventricular ejection fraction less than 40%.

The study found:

- Patients with lower cholesterol levels had a lower left ventricular ejection fraction.

- Patients with lower cholesterol levels had worse hemodynamic profiles.
- Patients with lower cholesterol levels had a higher New York Heart Association class.
- Patients with lower cholesterol died earlier.
- Patients with lower cholesterol had an increased risk of urgent transplant.

The study shows that low cholesterol levels are strongly associated with increased mortality in patients with nonischemic, systolic heart failure.

Paper 48
High cholesterol is a marker for longevity

Kalantar-Zadeh K et al Risk factor
paradox in wasting diseases.
Current Opinion in Clinical Nutrition &
Metabolic Care. 2007 Jul; 10(4) : 433-42

Professor Kamyar Kalantar-Zadeh is an American physician doing research in nephrology, nutrition, and epidemiology.

Kalantar-Zadeh reviewed the literature concerning cholesterol levels and disease and found that having high cholesterol leads to higher survival rates in people with chronic kidney disease, chronic heart failure, chronic obstructive lung disease, cancer, AIDS, rheumatoid arthritis, and in the elderly.

Paper 49
For each 1-mmol/L (38mg/dL) decrease in cholesterol levels, heart failure patients have a 26% increase in mortality risk

Smetanina IN et al Cholesterol and glucose levels
belong to independent predictors of death and
hospitalisations in patients with chronic systolic
heart failure. *Kardiologiia*. 2007; 47(8) : 12-6

This Russian study of 130 patients with systolic chronic heart failure was designed to elucidate the relationship of cholesterol levels with the number of deaths and hospitalisations of the patients for heart failure worsening over a 1.4 year period. Average age of the patients was 65 years.

The researchers found:

- Those patients who died or were hospitalised for worsening heart failure had lower cholesterol rates than those who remained healthy.
- For each 1-mmol/L (38mg/dL) decrease in cholesterol levels, patients had a 26% increase of mortality risk.
- Patients with cholesterol levels less than 4.0 mmol/L (154mg/dL) were at higher risk of death or been hospitalised for worsening heart failure.
- Patients with cholesterol levels less than 4.0 mmol/L (154mg/dL) had significantly reduced survival rates.

The findings of the study indicate that patients with heart failure are more likely to die or need hospital treatment if they have low cholesterol levels.

Paper 50
A 10ml INCREASE in cholesterol levels
are associated with a 4% DECREASED
risk of mortality from heart failure

Horwich TB Cholesterol levels and in-hospital mortality
in patients with acute decompensated heart failure.
American Heart Journal. Volume 156, Issue 6,
Pages 1170-1176 December 2008

Dr Tamara B Horwich headed the team in this study. She practices in Cardiovascular Disease and Internal Medicine.

The Get With the Guidelines–Heart Failure registry collects data on patients hospitalised with heart failure. Dr. Horwich and her researchers analysed data for over 2 years on 17,791 patients admitted between January 2005 and June 2007 at 236 participating hospitals who had their cholesterol levels recorded. 46% of the patients were on statins.

Dr Horwich discovered that each 10ml INCREASE in cholesterol level was associated with a 4% DECREASED risk of in-hospital mortality from heart failure.

Paper 51
Low cholesterol levels are associated with higher death rates in stroke, heart failure, and cancer

Nago N et al Low cholesterol is associated
with mortality from stroke, heart disease,
and cancer: the Jichi Medical School
Cohort Study. *Journal of Epidemiology.* 2011; 21(1) : 67-74

This Japanese study of 12,334 healthy adults aged 40 to 69 years investigated the relationship between low cholesterol and mortality and examined whether that relationship differs with respect to cause of death.

The study found:

- Those with the lowest cholesterol (under 4.14mmol/L - 160mg/dL) had around a 50% higher death rate than those with cholesterol up to 5.17mmol/L - 200mg/dL. High cholesterol (above 6.21mmol/L - 240mg/dL) was not a risk factor.
- The risk of death in the lowest cholesterol group for hemorrhagic stroke, heart failure (excluding myocardial infarction), and cancer mortality was significantly higher than those of the moderate cholesterol group, for each cause of death.

The information from this study pinpoints that low cholesterol is related to high mortality.

Paper 52
High cholesterol levels are associated with a 22% DECREASE in stroke incidence

Hamer M et al Comparison of risk factors for fatal stroke and ischemic heart disease: A prospective follow-up of the health survey for England. *Atherosclerosis.*
2011 Dec; 219(2) : 807-10

Dr Mark Hamer an expert In Cardiovascular Medicine, University College London compared risk factors for stroke and ischemic heart disease in 82,380 participants over a ten-year period (average age 55.4 years) who had no history of cardiovascular diseases.

Dr Hamer found:

- High total cholesterol levels had no bearing on heart disease rates.

- High total cholesterol levels were associated with a 22% decrease in stroke incidence.

More evidence from an expert that shows high cholesterol levels may in fact offer protection from cardiovascular diseases.

Paper 53
The higher your cholesterol
levels - the longer you live!

Petursson H et al Is the use of cholesterol in mortality risk algorithms in clinical guidelines valid? Ten years prospective data from the Norwegian HUNT 2 study.
Journal of Evaluation in Clinical Practice.
2012 Feb; 18(1) : 159-68

Halfdan Petursson is an Icelandic medical doctor whose research field is prevention of cardiovascular disease.

In this study of ten years of duration, Dr Petursson and his research team investigated if cholesterol levels are a risk factor for mortality in 52,087 individuals (24,235 men and 27,852 women) aged 20–74 years and free from known cardiovascular disease at the start of the study.

After analysing ten years of data Dr Petursson found:

- Compared with women whose cholesterol was under 5.0 mmol/l (193 mg/dl), those with a reading over 7.0 mmol/l (270 mg/dl) enjoyed a 28% reduction of death.
- Compared with men whose cholesterol was under 5.0 mmol/l (193 mg/dl), those with a reading over

7.0 mmol/l (270 mg/dl) enjoyed a 11% reduction of death.

- Compared with women whose cholesterol was under 5.0 mmol/l (193 mg/dl), those with a reading over 7.0 mmol/l (270 mg/dl) enjoyed a 26% reduction of cardiovascular diseases.
- Compared with men whose cholesterol was under 5.0 mmol/l (193 mg/dl), those with a reading up to 5.9 mmol/l (228 mg/dl) enjoyed a 20% reduction of cardiovascular diseases.

The study shows if you have cholesterol levels above 5.0 mmol/l (193 mg/dl), you will have less risk of heart disease and you will live longer.

Dr Petursson concluded; "the clinical and public health recommendations regarding the 'dangers' of cholesterol should be revised. This is especially true for women, for whom moderately elevated cholesterol (by current standards) may prove to be not only harmless but even bene?cial."

Paper 54
High HDL cholesterol gives protection from heart attacks

Goldbourt U et al High density lipoprotein cholesterol and incidence of coronary heart disease — the Israeli Ischemic Heart Disease Study. *American Journal of Epidemiology.* 1979 Mar; 109(3) : 296-308

Professor Uri Goldbourt holds a position at the Division of Epidemiology and Preventive Medicine, Sackler Medical Faculty, Tel Aviv University, Israel and was also a founding member and first chairperson of the Working group on cardiovascular Epidemiology and Preventive cardiology of the Israel heart Association in 1997.

In this paper Professor Goldbourt investigated the association between high density lipoprotein (HDL) cholesterol and coronary heart disease incidence over a five year period in 6,500 Israeli men aged over fifty.

Professor Goldbourt found that the higher your HDL cholesterol values, the less likely you are to have a heart attack, especially if you are a male over 50.

Eating a high percentage of dietary fat increases HDL cholesterol *(see papers 21, 30)*.

Paper 55
Association of low levels of HDL and
HDL2 cholesterol with heart disease

Laakso M et al Association of low HDL and HDL2 cholesterol with coronary heart disease in noninsulin-dependent diabetics. *Arteriosclerosis.*
1985 Nov-Dec; 5(6) : 653-8

The Cholesterol lipoproteins (HDL & HDL2) were measured by Dr Markku Laakso from Kuopio University Central Hospital Finland in 139 men and 145 women who were type two diabetics aged 45 to 64 years. Of these, 27 men and 16 women had had a previous definite heart attack.

The study found that:

- Those who had suffered a heart attack showed lower values of HDL and HDL2 cholesterol concentrations than those without a previous heart attack.

- Those who had suffered a heart attack showed lower values of HDL and HDL2 cholesterol concentrations than those without any symptoms or electrocardiographic signs of coronary heart disease.

The relationship between low levels of HDL & HDL2 cholesterol, and heart disease was evident in both sexes, but it was particularly strong among males.

Diets high in saturated fat can raise beneficial HDL cholesterol *(see paper 32)*.

Paper 56
Low HDL cholesterol and increased heart disease

Luc G et al Value of HDL cholesterol, apolipoprotein A-I, lipoprotein A-I, and lipoprotein A-I/A-II in prediction of coronary heart disease: the PRIME Study. Prospective Epidemiological Study of Myocardial Infarction. *Arteriosclerosis, Thrombosis, and Vascular Biology.* 2002 Jul 1; 22(7) : 1155-61

Apolipoprotein A-I is the major protein component of high-density lipoprotein (HDL) cholesterol. Lipoprotein A-I and lipoprotein A-I:A-II are constituents of Apolipoprotein A-I.

This study, based at the University of Lille, examined the association between the incidence of coronary heart disease and levels of four constituents of high-density lipoprotein (HDL) cholesterol in 9,073 French and Northern Irish men over a five-year period.

The four constituents of HDL cholesterol measured were:

- HDL cholesterol
- apolipoprotein A-I (apoA-I)
- lipoprotein A-I
- lipoprotein A-I:A-II

The study found:

- All four HDL cholesterol types levels were lower in coronary heart disease patients than in coronary heart disease-free subjects.
- Low levels of apolipoprotein A-I (apoA-I) were a particularly strong predictor of heart disease.

The paper illustrates how low levels of HDL cholesterol and especially low levels of apolipoprotein A-I (apoA-I) are a strong predictor of heart disease.

The most effective dietary way to raise HDL cholesterol is to consume a diet rich in saturated fat *(see papers 21, 30, 32, 37)*.

Paper 57
Low HDL cholesterol increases
coronary heart disease death in the elderly

Li JZ et al Apparent protective effect of high-density lipoprotein against coronary heart disease in the elderly.
Chinese Medical Journal. 2004 Apr; 117(4) : 511-5

This study was designed to evaluate the relationship between high-density lipoprotein cholesterol (HDL-C) levels and heart attack and coronary heart disease death and to explore the protective effect of HDL-C against heart disease in the elderly Chinese. The study included 1,211 retirees (92% males, average age 70) and lasted just over 11 years.

According to their HDL-C levels, subjects were divided into three groups and the differences in incidence of heart attack and heart disease death in each group were analysed. The groups were:

- ○ Low HDL-C (less than 1.03 mmol/L or 40mg/dL).
- ○ Medium HDL-C (or normal, 1.03 - 1.56 mmol/L or 40mg/dL - 60mg/dL).
- ○ High HDL-C (more than 1.56 mmol/L or 60mg/dL).

The study discovered:

- Heart attack occurrence and heart disease death in the normal HDL-C group was lower than in the low HDL-C group by 40% and 53% respectively.
- Heart attack occurrence and heart disease death in the high HDL-C group was lower than in the normal HDL-C group by 56% and 50% respectively.

The paper concludes that low HDL cholesterol is protective against heart attacks and Coronary Heart Disease death in the elderly; also high HDL cholesterol has significant protective effect against coronary artery disease.

HDL cholesterol can be increased by a high fat diet *(see papers 21, 28)*.

Paper 58
The "bad" low-density lipoprotein
(LDL) cholesterol levels have
NO association with heart disease rates

Elis A et al HDL-C Levels and Revascularisation
Procedures in Coronary Heart Disease Patients
Treated With Statins to Target LDL-C Levels.
Clinical Cardiology. 2011 Sep; 34(9) : 572-6

This Israeli study of 909 male patients investigated the relationship of high-density lipoprotein (HDL) cholesterol levels with revascularisation procedures in men whose LDL levels had been reduced to under 100 mg/dL by statin use.

Revascularisation is a surgical procedure for the provision of a new, additional, or augmented blood supply to a body part or organ:

- The study found the men who had the lowest HDL cholesterol had 24.2% more revascularisation procedures than the men who had the highest HDL cholesterol.
- All the men had been receiving statins to lower their LDL cholesterol. The statins had been successful in lowering their LDL-C to under 100mg/dL. This did not make any difference to whether they had cardiovascular problems or not.
- What did make a difference was the HDL-C levels. The higher the HDL-C, the less cardiovascular

problems occurred. Guess what is the best diet to raise your HDL-C levels? A diet high in saturated fat *(see paper 21)*.

This study shows that it is worthless to take statins to lower your LDL cholesterol, as it makes no difference to cardiovascular problems. However it does show that high HDL cholesterol levels offer protection from cardiovascular diseases, and we have seen that a high saturated fat diet increase HDL cholesterol more than any other type of food.

One explanation for the results of this study is the men who had the highest HDL cholesterol may have been consuming a diet high in saturated fat, which would firstly account for the high HDL cholesterol.

Secondly, high saturated fat diets are associated with lowering the amount of small and dense "bad" pattern B type of low-density lipoprotein (LDL) cholesterol to the more "heart friendly" large and fluffy type A *(see paper 91)*. So the men with the higher HDL cholesterol probably also had the healthier type A LDL cholesterol, which again may explain their lower rates of revascularisation procedures.

Paper 59
Saturated fat can help to lower
the rates of heart disease

Mora S et al Association of high-density lipoprotein cholesterol with incident cardiovascular events in women, by low-density lipoprotein cholesterol and apolipoprotein b100 levels: a cohort study. *Annals of Internal Medicine.* 2011 Dec 6; 155(11) :742-50

Dr Samia Mora who is an assistant professor of medicine at Harvard Medical School, headed this study where 26,861 initially healthy women, aged 45 years or older at the start of the study, were followed for approximately 11 years to determine the association between high density lipoprotein (HDL) cholesterol or apolipoprotein A-I levels and cardiovascular disease across a range of low density lipoprotein (LDL) cholesterol levels.

The study found:

- Those with the lowest levels of high density lipoprotein (HDL) cholesterol had a 119% increased risk of cardiovascular disease compared to those with the highest high density lipoprotein (HDL) cholesterol.
- Those with the lowest apolipoprotein A-I levels had a 58% increased risk of cardiovascular disease compared to those with the highest apolipoprotein A-I levels.
- The above associations were found for high-density lipoprotein (HDL) cholesterol with coronary events among women with a range of low density lipoprotein (LDL) cholesterol levels.

Similar to *paper 58* in men, this study of women shows that high levels of high-density lipoprotein (HDL) cholesterol are associated with lower rates of cardiovascular disease, no matter what the levels of low density lipoprotein (LDL) cholesterol are.

The best way to raise your high-density lipoprotein (HDL) cholesterol levels is to consume a diet rich in saturated fat *(see papers 21, 32, 37).*

I hope the studies in this chapter have given you an insight into the role of cholesterol levels and disease.

The data shows how low cholesterol levels are associated with more heart attacks and strokes.

Many studies report how the lower your cholesterol is, the more likely you are to die of heart failure.

A thorough examination of the scientific literature revealed that LOW cholesterol levels are linked to earlier death in the elderly and to many diseases and conditions such as; kidney disease, lung disease, heart failure, cancer, AIDS, rheumatoid arthritis, and in accidents, violent deaths and suicide.

High levels of the "good" high-density lipoprotein (HDL) cholesterol have been shown to be strongly associated with lower rates of heart disease, and the best way to elevate your "good" HDL cholesterol levels is to eat a diet high in saturated fat.

However the two biggest revelations that this chapter has brought to light is that high cholesterol levels are associated with lower rates of cardiovascular disease and that having a higher cholesterol level means you will probably live longer.

So to answer the three questions from the start of the chapter;

What is a "dangerously high" cholesterol level?
The question we should be asking is; what is a "dangerously low" cholesterol level?

Should we all be on cholesterol lowering medication?

Considering that lower cholesterol levels are associated with higher rates of cardiovascular disease, kidney disease, lung disease, heart failure, cancer, AIDS, rheumatoid arthritis, and in accidents, violent deaths and suicide, the answer is a resounding NO!

Should we be trying to lower our cholesterol in the first place?

For the same reasons as the previous question the answer again is an emphatic NO!

What we should be doing is increasing our dietary saturated fat intake because:

- Saturated fat raises our "heart friendly" high-density lipoprotein (HDL) cholesterol levels.
- Saturated fat changes our low-density lipoprotein (LDL) cholesterol from the "dangerous" small and dense pattern B, to the relatively benign light and fluffy pattern A.

To sum up the scientific evidence from this chapter: Having higher cholesterol means you are at LESS risk from cardiovascular disease (and many other diseases) and you will live longer.

So if cholesterol and saturated fat do not cause heart disease, what does cause heart disease?

The scientific papers in the next chapter will undertake to answer that question.

CHAPTER 4

What does cause
heart disease?

The previous chapters have established that cholesterol and saturated fat are heart protective.

What then are we doing different from a time when there was very little heart disease, to the present day when it seems heart disease is almost compulsory?

Are we told the correct dietary advice?

This chapter will take you through the studies that point the finger of blame as to the factors that do cause heart disease.

Paper 60
High carbohydrate diets are associated
with an increase in incidence
of coronary artery disease
Coulston A et al Plasma glucose, insulin and lipid responses
to high-carbohydrate low-fat diets in normal humans.
Metabolism. Volume 32, Issue 1, January 1983, Pages 52-56

This Stanford University study investigated the effects of two diets in 11 healthy volunteers over 10 days to ascertain the diets effects on insulin, triglyceride (TG) and high-density lipoprotein (HDL)-cholesterol concentrations were analysed. One diet had 40% carbohydrate of calories (Lower Carb), the other at 60% carbohydrate of calories (Higher Carb).

The researchers found:

- (Bad) Triglyceride levels *(see paper 88)* were increased on the higher carb diet.
- (Bad) Insulin levels were *(see paper 78)* increased on the higher carb diet.
- (Good) HDL-cholesterol concentrations *(see paper 56)* were decreased on the higher carb diet.

The study leader, Ann Coulston concluded: *"These results indicate that high-carbohydrate diets lead to changes in insulin, triglycerides, and HDL-cholesterol concentrations which have been associated with an increase in incidence of coronary artery disease".*

Paper 61
Study of over 1 million men shows that eating a low-fat, vegetable based diet gives a seven-fold increased risk of heart disease

Malhorta SL et al Epidemiology of Ischamic Heart Disease in India with Special Reference to Causation. *British Heart Journal* 1967, 29, 895

This study, published in the prestigious *British Heart Journal,* included 1,150,000 railway workers between the ages of 18-55 years serving on the railways in different parts of India.

- In the north the consumption of fats, (most of which are animal fats), is 19 times more than in the south. Heart disease is seven times less in the north than in the south.
- Moreover, while the milk fats eaten in the north have a preponderance of saturated fatty acids, the seed oils used in the south are mainly composed of unsaturated fatty acids.
- Vegetable consumption is around 33% lower in the north than in the south.

This massive study of over 1 million men shows that eating a low-fat, vegetable based diet gives a seven-fold increased risk of heart disease compared to a diet 19 times richer in fat.

Paper 62
High carbohydrate diet leads to adverse health effects

Garg A et al Effects of Varying Carbohydrate Content of Diet in Patients With Non-Insulin Dependent Diabetes Mellitus. *Journal of the American Medical Association.* 1994; 271 : 1421-1428

The objective of the study was to determine the effects of a diet high in carbohydrate versus a diet high in fat on blood sugar and cholesterol values in patients with diabetes. 42 patients were involved in the study and they received a diet of either:

- 55% carbohydrate, 30% fat (high carbohydrate diet).
- 40% carbohydrate 45% fat (high fat diet).

Dr Abhimanyu Garg who headed the study found:

- The high carbohydrate diet increased (bad) triglyceride levels by 24% compared to the high fat diet.
- The high carbohydrate diet increased (bad) very low-density lipoprotein cholesterol (VLDL) levels by 23% compared to the high fat diet.
- The high carbohydrate diet increased (bad) daylong insulin levels by 9% compared to the high fat diet.

Dr Garg aptly comments that the *high carbohydrate diet "may not be desirable"* because:

High triglyceride levels are associated with non-alcoholic fatty liver disease, heart failure, diabetes and heart disease *(see paper 88).*

High, very low-density lipoprotein cholesterol (VLDL) levels are associated with diabetes, heart disease and stroke *(see paper 92).*

High insulin levels are associated with heart disease *(see paper 78)*, cancer, high blood pressure and obesity.

Paper 63
Diets high in carbohydrates which have a high glycemic load, increase heart disease risk by 98%

Liu S et al A prospective study of dietary glycemic load, carbohydrate intake, and risk of coronary heart disease in US women. *American Journal of Clinical Nutrition.* 2000 Jun; 71(6) : 1455-61

The objective of this Harvard University study was to evaluate the relationship between the amount and type of dietary carbohydrates with the risk of heart disease. 75,521 women aged 38-63 years with no previous diagnosis of diabetes or cardiovascular diseases were followed for 10 years. (729,472 person-years).

After 10 years of data the researchers found:

- The women who consumed foods with the highest glycemic load had a 98% increased risk of heart disease.
- Women who consumed foods with the highest carbohydrate content had a 23% increased risk of heart disease.
- Women with high dietary glycemic loads consumed more carbohydrates, dietary fibre and cereal fibre, but had lower intakes of fats, cholesterol and proteins, than did women with low glycemic loads.
- The two most important contributors to dietary glycemic load in this population were mashed or baked potatoes and cold breakfast cereals.

Foods with a high glycemic load include:

cornflakes, coco pops, special K, grape nuts, bagels, dried dates, rice, buckwheat, macaroni, spaghetti and potatoes.

The results of this study show that diets high in carbohydrates that have a high glycemic load are associated with a 98% increase in heart disease.

Paper 64
Low fat diets in children may
lead to clogged arteries in adulthood

Lifshitz F et al Considerations about dietary
fat restrictions for children. *Journal of Nutrition.*
1996 Apr; 126(4 Suppl) : 1031S-41S

This paper, penned by Dr Fima Lifshitz MD who is a
Pediatric Endocrinologist and has over 50 years
experience and background in medicine, examined the
evidence regarding the appropriateness of low fat diets
for children.

The review found:

- There is no data demonstrating any beneficial
  effects of low fat diets starting in childhood for
  children.
- Dietary fat restriction in early life has not been
  shown to reduce disease incidence.
- Low fat diets in children are linked with
  suboptimal growth and development. Recent
  studies have shown an association between short
  stature and/or nutritional status and deficiencies
  in intrauterine and early life with coronary artery
  disease in adulthood.
- Low fat diets may lower (the good) high-density
  lipoprotein (HDL) cholesterol levels.
- Low fat diets may lower total cholesterol levels.
  However low total cholesterol levels may be
  associated with increased mortality, including
  deaths due to accidents, which is most important in
  children.

○ Problems of associated psychological consequences, family conflicts and cost should not be ignored while implementing a low fat diet.

Lifshitz notes many qualities of dietary fat and that it is an essential component of a well-balanced diet:

- In addition to being an efficient energy source, fat, compared with other macronutrients, has the advantage of carrying more energy in a smaller volume. This is of vital importance for children who have limited intake capacity but extraordinary energy needs.
- Fat and cholesterol constitute an essential structural element of the cellular membranes.
- Essential fats are vital for the central nervous system including visual development and intelligence.
- High blood pressure and clogged arteries may be among the consequences of insufficient essential fats. Therefore, low fat diets that could lead to essential fat deficiencies could be detrimental rather than beneficial.
- Fat is also necessary as a vehicle to carry the fat soluble vitamins (A,D,E,K). Numerous studies have shown that low fat diets lead to vitamin and mineral deficiencies either because they are not consumed in adequate amounts in restricted diets or their absorption is decreased when fat intake is inadequate.
- Low cholesterol diets may lead to hormonal problems as all adrenocortical hormones (such as aldosterone and cortisol) are synthesised from cholesterol.

Dr Lifshitz found that low fat diets may be detrimental to children's health for a myriad of reasons, including a link to heart disease in adulthood.

Paper 65
Low fat/high carbohydrate diets are associated with higher heart disease risk

Parks EJ et al Effects of a low-fat, high-carbohydrate diet on VLDL-triglyceride assembly, production, and clearance. *Journal of Clinical Investigation.* 1999 Oct; 104(8) : 1087-96

This study, headed by Dr Elizabeth Parks, investigated the effects of a low-fat, high-carbohydrate (LF/HC diet) on (heart harmful) triglyceride levels *(see paper 88)* and other heart disease risk markers. In this trial volunteers consumed a low fat diet (15% fat) for a five-week period.

By the end of the study the low-fat, high-carbohydrate (LF/HC) diet produced the following:

- The LF/HC diet resulted in a 60% elevation in (bad) triglyceride concentrations.
- The LF/HC diet resulted in a 37% reduction in very low density lipoprotein-triglyceride (VLDL-TG clearance) -which means higher levels of the (bad) VLDL-TG.
- The LF/HC diet resulted in an 18% reduction in whole-body fat oxidation -which means the body burns fat more slowly and makes you fatter.
- The LF/HC diet resulted in significant elevations in fasting apo B-48 concentrations. Apo B-48 concentrations are a marker for chylomicron

remnants *(see paper 89)*, which are associated with heart disease *(see paper 86)*.

The results of this trial by Dr Parks suggest that low-fat, high-carbohydrate diets may increase the risk of heart disease.

Paper 66
Heart disease risk is increased
by a high carbohydrate diet

Koutsari C et al Exercise prevents the accumulation of triglyceride-rich lipoproteins and their remnants seen when changing to a high-carbohydrate diet. *Arteriosclerosis, Thrombosis, and Vascular Biology.* 2001 Sep; 21(9) : 1520-5

Levels of the unhealthy triglycerides and apolipoprotein B-48 and apolipoprotein B-100 were measured in healthy postmenopausal women aged 51 to 66 years after consuming either a high fat diet or a high carbohydrate diet in this UK study.

The diets were either:

○ A high fat diet (35%, 50%, and 15% energy from carbohydrate, fat, and protein, respectively).
○ A high carbohydrate diet (corresponding values 70%, 15%, and 15%).

The study revealed that:

• (Bad) Triglyceride levels were higher after the high-carbohydrate diet than after the low-carbohydrate diet.

- Concentrations of (the bad) apolipoproteins apoB-48 and apoB-100 were significantly higher after the high-carbohydrate diet.

High triglyceride and apolipoprotein B levels may lead to heart disease *(see papers 88, 89)*.

Paper 67
Low fat diets do not provide adequate nutrition and increase heart disease risk factors

Meksawan K et al Effect of Low and High Fat Diets on Nutrient Intakes and Selected Cardiovascular Risk Factors in Sedentary Men and Women. *Journal of the American College of Nutrition.* Vol. 23, No. 2, 131-140 2004

Researchers at the State University of New York conducted a study to determine the effects of a low fat diet (19% fat) and a high fat diet (50% fat) on the nutritional status and cardiovascular risk factors in healthy individuals over a three-week period.

Kulwara Meksawan, who led the study, reported:

- Consumptions of essential fatty acids, vitamin E and zinc were improved in the high fat diet.
- Compared with the 50% fat diet, subjects consuming the 19% fat diet had significantly lower levels of the beneficial high-density lipoprotein (HDL) cholesterol and apolipoprotein A1 (ApoA1).

The paper concludes that a low fat diet (19%) may not provide sufficient calories, essential fatty acids, and some micronutrients (especially vitamin E and zinc) for healthy individuals, and it also lowered the beneficial ApoA1 and HDL cholesterol *(see papers 56, 59).* Increasing fat intake to 50% of calories improved nutritional status, and led to higher HDL cholesterol values.

Paper 68
In postmenopausal women, carbohydrate intake is associated with a progression of heart disease

Mozaffarian D et al Dietary fats, carbohydrate, and progression of coronary atherosclerosis in postmenopausal women. *American Journal of Clinical Nutrition.* Vol. 80, No. 5, 1175-1184

Dr Dariush Mozaffarian is an Associate Professor in the Department of Epidemiology at the Harvard School of Public Health. His area of expertise lies in the effects of diet on cardiovascular diseases.

The objective of this study, led by Dr Mozaffarian, was to investigate associations between dietary fat and carbohydrate and the amount of blockage in the arteries among postmenopausal women.

2,243 coronary artery diameters were measured over 3.1 years in 235 postmenopausal women with established coronary heart disease.

The study found:

- Those with the highest saturated fat intake had no change in their arteries.

- Those with the lowest saturated fat intake had the biggest increase in blockages in their arteries.
- Higher carbohydrate consumption was associated with an increase in blocked arteries.
- Polyunsaturated fat consumption was associated with an increase in blocked arteries, when it replaced other fats in the diet.

Dr Mozaffarian found in postmenopausal women, a greater saturated fat intake is associated with less progression of heart disease, whereas carbohydrate intake is associated with a greater progression of heart disease.

Paper 69
Low fat, high carbohydrate diets increase the risk of heart disease

Min-Jeong Shin et al Increased plasma concentrations of lipoprotein (a) during a low-fat, high-carbohydrate diet are associated with increased plasma concentrations of apolipoprotein C-III bound to apolipoprotein B–containing lipoproteins. *American Journal of Clinical Nutrition.* Vol. 85, No. 6, 1527-1532, June 2007

Min-Jeong Shin, who headed the team in this study, is an assistant professor in the Department of Food and Nutrition at Korea University. She specialises in lifestyle modification in the prevention of heart disease.

In this study 140 healthy men consumed either high fat/low carbohydrate diet or a low fat/high carbohydrate diets to measure the effects each diet had on heart disease risk factors.

The diets lasted for four weeks and comprised of:

- High-fat, low-carbohydrate diet (HFLC diet 40% fat, 45% carbohydrate).
- Low-fat, high carbohydrate diet (LFHC diet 20% fat, 65% carbohydrate).

Professor Shin found that concentrations of Lipoprotein (a), triglycerides, Apolipoprotein B, Apolipoprotein C-III were all higher on the low fat, high carbohydrate diet compared to a high fat, low carbohydrate diet.

All four of these values on the low fat, high carbohydrate diet indicate an increased risk of heart disease:

- Lipoprotein (a) *(see paper 85)*.
- Triglycerides *(see paper 88)*.
- Apolipoprotein B *(see paper 89)*.
- Apolipoprotein C-III *(see paper 90)*.

Paper 70
Increase in heart disease risk factors on a low fat high carbohydrate diet

Faghihnia N et al Changes in lipoprotein (a), oxidised phospholipids, and LDL sub-classes with a low-fat high-carbohydrate diet. *Journal of Lipid Research*. 51, 3324-3330 November 2010

This study, based at the University of California, looked at how a high-fat, low-carbohydrate (HFLC) diet and a low-fat, high carbohydrate diet (LFHC) affected different types of cholesterol in 63 healthy subjects over a four week period.

The study found that:

- The (bad) Lipoprotein (a) levels *(see paper 84)* increased on the low fat/high carbohydrate diet compared to the high fat/low carbohydrate diet.
- The (bad) apolipoprotein (apo)B levels *(see paper 89)* increased on the low fat/high carbohydrate diet compared to the high fat/low carbohydrate diet.
- Low-density lipoprotein (LDL) cholesterol particle size decreased to a (bad) smaller size *(see papers 87, 91)* on the low fat/high carbohydrate diet compared to the high fat/low carbohydrate diet.
- The total number of (bad) very low-density lipoprotein (VLDL) particles *(see paper 90)* increased on the low fat/high carbohydrate diet compared to the high fat/low carbohydrate diet.

The changes in the above cholesterol levels by the low fat/high carbohydrate diet are associated with an increased heart disease risk.

Paper 71
Vegetable oils implicated
in increased death rates

Christakis G Effect of the Anti-Coronary Club Program on Coronary Heart Disease Risk-Factor Status. *Journal of the American Medical Association.* Nov 7 1966 198 (6) 597-604

In this study, published in the prestigious *Journal of the American Medical Association,* 814 men were put on a diet where they greatly reduced their animal fat consumption, which was replaced by a "Prudent Diet" of polyunsaturated vegetable oils. 463 other men continued to eat their normal higher animal fat diet.

- After four years the men in the *"prudent"* group had lowered their cholesterol by 35mg/100ml and the men in the *"normal"* group had unchanged cholesterol.
- There were a total of 27 deaths in the *"vegetable oil, prudent"* group and only six deaths (none of which were from heart disease) in the *"high animal fat, normal"* group.

This four and a half fold increase in death rates in men who consumed a high vegetable oil diet is confirmed when analysing the rates of heart disease and the consumption rates of vegetable oil and animal fats since 1910.

In 1910 the death rates from heart attacks were virtually nonexistent, whereas now heart disease is the world's number one killer.

Since that time vegetable oil consumption has increased five fold and the levels of dietary saturated animal fats has actually declined.

These figures show that saturated animal fats cannot be the cause of heart disease, whereas a massive increase in the consumption of vegetable oils has coincided with heart disease becoming the leading cause of death in the world today.

Paper 72
Margarine increases the risk of heart disease

Fumeron F et al Lowering of HDL2-cholesterol
and lipoprotein A-I particle levels by increasing
the ratio of polyunsaturated to saturated fatty acids.
American Journal of Clinical Nutrition. Vol 53, 655-659

Dr F Fumeron who led this French study, notes that the protective role of high-density lipoprotein cholesterol (HDL) against heart disease has been attributed to high densities of the HDL sub-fractions HDL2 and apolipoprotein A-I (apoA-1).

The study investigated the effect of a high ratio of polyunsaturated to saturated fatty acids on these sub-fractions in a group of 36 young adult males. Two diets were consumed at the subjects' homes for three weeks each.

The diets were identical apart from one was supplemented with butter and the other with margarine as follows:

- ○ 70 g butter (LOW polyunsaturated fat/saturated fat ratio) *High saturated fat diet.*
- ○ 70 g sunflower margarine (HIGH polyunsaturated fat/saturated fat ratio) *High polyunsaturated fat diet.*
- • Significant decreases in the protective sub-fractions of HDL; HDL2, and apoA-1 were observed in the margarine, *high polyunsaturated fat diet* compared to the *high saturated fat diet.*

The study reveals that the high polyunsaturated fat diet (margarine) diminishes the two highly protective HDL cholesterol sub fractions, HDL2 and apoA-1, which could be detrimental and increase the risk of heart disease.

Margarine's heart disease causing characteristics are understandable when its production methods are scrutinized.

Margarine is made from the cheapest (highly contaminated with pesticides and often genetically modified) vegetable oils, such as soy, safflower seeds, cottonseed, soy beans, sunflower seeds and canola.

These oils are extracted from the seeds using high temperature and high pressure production methods. Unfortunately this turns the oils rancid, which can lead to health problems such as cell damage, premature aging and many other problems.

A solvent called hexane is used to make sure all the oil is extracted. Hexane is known to cause cancer.

Once the oil is extracted it is steam cleaned which destroys all the vitamins, but does not remove all the pesticides and hexane.

Toxic catalysts such as nickel are then mixed into the oil to speed up the hydrogenation procedure, which of course produces the dangerous "trans fats".

The margarine is now a grey coloured smelly lump of grease.

Soapy emulsifiers are mixed in to remove the lumps and the grease is deodorized under high temperature and high pressure. To finish the cleaning the grease is bleached to remove the grey colour.

The manufacturing process so far has completely stripped the product of all its natural vitamins, nutrients and flavours so a few synthetic vitamins and artificial flavours are mixed in.

A yellow colour is added, so it resembles butter.

This rancid mass is then marketed as a "health food".

Paper 73
Medium or high intake of margarine is associated with a 50% increased risk of a non-fatal heart attack

Tavani A et al Margarine intake and risk of non-fatal acute myocardial infarction in Italian women. *European Journal of Clinical Nutrition.* January 1997, Volume 51, Number 1, Pages 30-32

In this study Dr Alessandra Tavani and her researchers examined the relationship between margarine intake and nonfatal heart attacks in 429 Italian women, aged 18-74 years, in hospital with diagnosis of heart attack and 866 patients without heart disease.

- The study found that a medium or high intake of margarine was associated with a 50% increased risk of non-fatal heart attack.

The findings of this study are predictable when you analyse heart disease rates to butter and margarine consumption from the year 1909 onwards.

As noted *(see paper 71)*, heart disease rates were very low at the start of the 1900's. Now of course heart disease has been the biggest killer of people for decades.

Data shows that in 1909 butter consumption was 18 grams per person per day. In the same year the amount of margarine consumed was only two grams per person per day.

Figures for 1985 show butter consumption has plummeted by 360% and margarine consumption has shot up by 550%.

Again this data shows that butter (a saturated fat) cannot be the cause of the rise in heart disease, whereas the enormous rise in margarine consumption has mirrored the enormous rise in heart disease.

Paper 74
Margarine intake increases
the risk of heart disease

Gillman MW et al Margarine intake and
subsequent coronary heart disease in men.
Epidemiology. 1997 Mar; 8(2) : 144-9

This study, authored by Matthew Gillman who is a Professor in the Department of Nutrition at the Harvard School of Public Health, compared margarine and butter consumption on 832 men age 45-64 years and free of heart disease, with over 21 years of follow-up.

The study found that:

- For each increment of one teaspoon per day of margarine there was a 10% increase of heart disease over 21 years.

• Butter intake did not predict heart disease incidence.

Gillman concluded that the 21 year study offered support to the hypothesis that margarine intake increases the risk of coronary heart disease.

It's unsurprising that margarine causes an increase in heart disease, because margarine is actually an industrially produced food commodity made with a long list of chemicals and additives.

Below is a list of all the ingredients in margarine:

Edible oils, edible fats, salt or potassium chloride, ascorbyl palmitate, butylated hydroxyanisole, phospholipids, tert-butylhydroquinone, mono-and di-glycerides of fat-forming fatty acids, disodium guanylate, diacetyltartaric and fatty acid esters of glycerol, Propyl, octyl or dodecyl gallate (or mixtures thereof), tocopherols, propylene glycol mono- and di-esters, sucrose esters of fatty acids, curcumin, annatto extracts, tartaric acid, 3,5,trimethylhexanal, β-apo-carotenoic acid methyl or ethyl ester, skim milk powder, xanthophylls and canthaxanthin.

Paper 75
Margarine damages the lining of blood vessels

Hennig B et al PCB-induced oxidative stress
in endothelial cells: modulation by nutrients.
*International Journal of Hygiene and
Environmental Health.* 2002 Mar; 205(1-2) : 95-102

The lead researcher in this paper is Dr Bernhard Hennig, who is professor of nutrition and toxicology with the University of Kentucky.

From his research Dr Hennig found that polychlorinated biphenyls (PCBs) can damage the lining of blood vessels (endothelial dysfunction), which can lead to heart disease and that polyunsaturated omega-6 oils can increase this damage.

<u>List of the top 20 foods highest in Total Omega-6 polyunsaturated fat per 100-gram serving.</u>

1 Oil, vegetable safflower, salad or cooking, linoleic, (over 70%). Total Omega-6 fatty acids: 74615mg.

2 Oil, vegetable, grapeseed. Total Omega-6 fatty acids: 69591mg.

3 Oil, vegetable, sunflower, linoleic, (approx. 65%). Total Omega-6 fatty acids: 65702mg.

4 Oil, vegetable, poppyseed. Total Omega-6 fatty acids: 62391mg.

5 USDA Commodity Food, oil, vegetable, low saturated fat. Total Omega-6 fatty acids: 57724mg.

6 Oil, wheat germ. Total Omega-6 fatty acids: 54797mg.

7 Oil, vegetable, corn, industrial and retail, all purpose salad or cooking. Total Omega-6 fatty acids: 53510mg.

8 Oil, vegetable, walnut. Total Omega-6 fatty acids: 52894mg

9 Salad dressing, mayonnaise, soybean and safflower oil, with salt. Total Omega-6 fatty acids: 52002mg.

10 Oil, vegetable, cottonseed, salad or cooking. Total Omega-6 fatty acids: 51503mg.

11 Oil, vegetable, industrial, soy, refined, for woks and light frying. Total Omega-6 fatty acids: 51288mg.

12 Oil, vegetable, tomato seed. Total Omega-6 fatty acids: 50796mg.

13 Oil, soybean, salad or cooking. Total Omega-6 fatty acids: 50422mg.

14 USDA Commodity Food, oil, vegetable, soybean, refined. Total Omega-6 fatty acids: 50293mg.

15 Oil, cooking and salad, ENOVA, 80% diglycerides. Total Omega-6 fatty acids: 45937mg.

16 Oil, soybean, salad or cooking, (hydrogenated) and cottonseed. Total Omega-6 fatty acids: 45307mg.

17 Oil, sesame, salad or cooking. Total Omega-6 fatty acids: 41304mg.

18 Oil, vegetable, industrial, soy (partially hydrogenated) and soy (winterized), pourable clear fry. Total Omega-6 fatty acids: 40947mg.

19 Mayonnaise dressing, no cholesterol. Total Omega-6 fatty acids: 40567mg.

20 USDA Commodity Food, shortening, type III, creamy liquid, soybean and soybean (partially hydrogenated). Total Omega-6 fatty acids: 40204mg.

Most of the top 20 omega-6 foods are vegetable oils such as soy, sunflower and safflower which are extensively used in the manufacture of margarine.

Paper 76
Sunflower oil and olive oil increase
heart disease risk factors compared to butter

Mekki N et al Butter differs from olive oil and sunflower oil in its effects on postprandial lipemia and triacylglycerol-rich lipoproteins after single mixed meals in healthy young men. *Journal of Nutrition.* 2002 Dec; 132(12) : 3642-9

Nadia Mekki, the head researcher of the study, notes how excess triglyceride levels accumulated after meals are related to heart disease risk.

The goal of the study was to evaluate the effects of saturated fat (butter), monounsaturated fat (olive oil) or omega-6 polyunsaturated fat (sunflower oil) on post meal blood triglyceride and fat levels in healthy young men.

Mekki discovered:

- The two unsaturated oils (olive oil and sunflower oil, found in many margarines) induced a higher post meal rise in (bad) triglyceride and (bad) chylomicron levels than the butter meal.
- Circulating chylomicrons were smaller after the butter meal than after the two vegetable oil meals. (So they can be eliminated more easily)

Mekki concluded that consumption of butter results in lower triglyceride and chylomicron levels in the circulation of young men than consumption of olive or sunflower oils.

High triglycerides and chylomicrons levels are implicated in heart disease *(see papers 88, 86)*.

Thereby butter is more heart healthy than sunflower oil and olive oil.

Paper 77
Sunflower oil damages the blood vessels
Berry SE et al Impaired postprandial endothelial function depends on the type of fat consumed by healthy men.
Journal of Nutrition. 2008 Oct; 138(10) : 1910-4

This UK study, headed by Dr Sarah Berry, investigated the effects of saturated fat (butter) meals and monounsaturated fat (sunflower oil, found in many margarines) meals on the function of the blood vessels in 17 men.

Dr Berry found that:

- The rise in (bad) triglycerides *(see paper 88)* was 66% LESS after the butter meal than after the sunflower oil meal.
- After the sunflower oil meal there was a DECREASE in blood flow and an INCREASE in cell damage.
- After the butter meal there was NO change in blood flow and NO cell damage.

The study shows how sunflower oil damages the blood vessels, which may lead to heart disease.

Paper 78
High insulin levels linked to heart disease
Ducimetiere P et al Relationship of plasma insulin levels to the incidence of myocardial infarction and coronary heart disease mortality in a middle-aged population. *Diabetologia.* Volume 19, Number 3, 205-210

The study investigated the possible role of insulin levels as a risk factor of heart disease. The study included 7,246 non-diabetic, working men, aged 43–54 years, initially free from heart disease, and followed for 63 months on average.

Pierre Ducimetiere, the author of the study found that insulin levels were associated with heart disease and concluded: *"high insulin levels may constitute an independent risk factor for coronary heart disease complications in middle aged non-diabetic men".*

High insulin levels are caused by high carbohydrate diets *(see papers 60, 62).*

Paper 79
Vegan diet may lead to heart disease risk

Arnesen E et al Serum Total Homocysteine
and Coronary Heart Disease.
International Journal of Epidemiology.
Volume 24, Number 4 Pp. 704-709

In this Norwegian study the homocysteine levels of 21,826 subjects, aged 12–61 years were measured to investigate the relationship between homocysteine and heart disease.

- The study found that for each four µmol/l increase in homocysteine levels there was a 32% increased risk of heart disease.

Professor Egil Arnesen who headed the study concluded that high homocysteine levels are a risk factor for heart disease.

High homocysteine levels may be the result of B vitamin deficiencies caused by a vegetarian diet *(see paper 14).*

The best dietary sources of B vitamins are meat and poultry.

Paper 80
Soy consumption increases Lp(a),
an independent risk factor for heart disease

Nilausen K et al Lipoprotein (a) and dietary proteins:
casein lowers lipoprotein (a) concentrations as
compared with soy protein. *American Journal
of Clinical Nutrition.* Vol. 69, No. 3, 419-425, March 1999

The study was led by Dr Karin Nilausen of the University of Copenhagen School of Medicine who noted that lipoprotein (a) [Lp(a)], is an independent risk factor for coronary artery disease *(see papers 84, 85).*

The study compared the effects of dietary soy protein and casein on plasma Lp(a) concentrations. Men with normal cholesterol were studied initially while consuming their habitual, self-selected diets and then they consumed liquid-formula diets containing either casein or soy protein.

The study found:

- After 30 days Lp(a) decreased by an average of 50% after the casein diet as compared with concentrations after both the soy-protein and self-selected diets.
- Two weeks after subjects switched from the self-selected to the soy-protein diet, Lp(a) increased by 20%. In contrast, the switch to the casein diet caused a decrease in Lp(a) levels of 65%.

Dr Nilausen concluded: These findings indicate that soy protein may have an Lp(a)-raising effect which is an independent risk factor for heart disease.

Paper 81
High fat diets reduce dangerous
C-reactive protein levels by 52.6%

McAuley KA et al Comparison of high-fat and
high-protein diets with a high-carbohydrate
diet in insulin-resistant obese women.
Diabetologia. 2005 Jan; 48(1) : 8-16

High levels of C-reactive protein and triglycerides are
associated with an increased risk of heart disease *(see
paper 88).*

This New Zealand study investigated the effects of three
diets on diabetes and heart disease risk factors, such as
weight, triglyceride levels and C-reactive protein levels in
96 overweight insulin-resistant women.

The diets were either:

○ High-carbohydrate, high-fibre diet.
○ High-protein diet.
○ High-fat diet.

Dr Kirsten McAuley from the University of Otago who
headed the research team found:

• When compared with the high carbohydrate diet, the
high-fat and high-protein diets were shown to produce
significantly greater reductions in weight loss.
• When compared with the high carbohydrate
diet, the high-fat and high-protein diets were
shown to produce significantly greater reductions
in triglyceride levels.

- All diets reduced C-reactive protein levels. The high-carbohydrate diet reduced them by 14.8% and the high-protein diet by 17.3%. However, by far the largest decrease in the dangerous C-reactive protein levels was on the high-fat diet, with a 52.6% reduction.

This study reveals how a high fat diet is effective in reducing the risk of heart disease, with weight loss and the reduction of heart disease risk factors such as triglyceride and C-reactive protein levels.

Paper 82
Aspirin increases the risk
of heart disease and stroke

Belch J et al The prevention of progression of arterial disease and diabetes (POPADAD) trial: factorial randomised placebo controlled trial of aspirin and antioxidants in patients with diabetes and asymptomatic peripheral arterial disease. *British Medical Journal.* 2008; 337 : a1840

The objective of this Scottish study was to determine whether aspirin and antioxidant therapy are more effective than placebo in reducing the development of cardiovascular events in patients with diabetes and peripheral arterial disease. The study involved 1,276 patients aged 40 or more with diabetes who were assigned aspirin, antioxidants or placebo. Jill Belch, professor of vascular medicine from the University of Dundee led the study.

The study found;

- There was a 23% increased risk of coronary heart disease or stroke in those who took aspirin compared to those who did not take aspirin.

- There was a 21% increased risk of coronary heart disease or stroke in those who took antioxidants compared to those who did not take antioxidants.

This study demonstrated aspirin or antioxidants were ineffective at reducing the development of cardiovascular disease and in fact actually raised the risk of heart disease and stroke.

Paper 83
Appetite suppressant pills lead to a 28% higher risk of having a heart attack and a 36% higher risk of developing a stroke

James WPT et al Effect of Sibutramine on Cardiovascular Outcomes in Overweight and Obese Subjects.
New England Journal of Medicine. 363 :
905-917 September 2, 2010

Sibutramine, brand name Meridia is an appetite suppressant, a weight loss pill.

The study, published in the *New England Journal of Medicine,* lasted nearly three and a half years and involved 10,744 overweight or obese subjects, 55 years of age or older to assess the cardiovascular consequences of weight management with and without sibutramine. Patients were assigned either Meridia or a placebo.

The researchers report that:

- Those on Meridia had a 28% higher risk of a heart attack compared to placebo.
- Those on Meridia had a 36% higher risk of a stroke compared to placebo.

The results from this paper suggest ingesting appetite suppressant pills lead to higher rates of cardiovascular disease.

Paper 84
A high saturated fat diet
gives protection from heart disease

Rhoads GG et al Lp(a) Lipoprotein
as a Risk Factor for Myocardial Infarction.
Journal of the American Medical Association.
1986; 256 : 2540-2544

Professor Rhoads notes that lipoprotein (a) [Lp(a)] is structurally similar to low-density lipoprotein cholesterol (LDL), only it has an additional protein (the "little a") and is associated with heart disease.

To test the generalizability of this association, the study measured serum Lp(a) in 303 Hawaiian men of Japanese ancestry who had suffered a heart attack and in 408 others free from heart disease.

Professor Rhoads study revealed that men who had suffered a heart attack had 24% higher Lp(a) levels than those free from heart disease.

High saturated fat diets lower Lp(a) levels *(see papers 24, 70).*

Paper 85
High Lp(a) levels linked to heart
disease-Saturated fat lowers Lp(a) levels

Genest J et al Prevalence of lipoprotein (a) [Lp(a)]
excess in coronary artery disease.

American Journal of Cardiology. Volume 67,
Issue 13, 15 May 1991, Pages 1039-1045

Dr Jacques Genest from Tufts University notes that elevated levels of lipoprotein (a) [Lp(a)] have been associated with heart disease.

The purpose of the study was to determine the prevalence of Lp(a) excess in patients with heart disease.

Levels of Lp(a) were determined in 180 patients (150 men and 30 women) with heart disease before age 60 years, and in 459 control subjects free of cardiovascular disease.

- The study revealed that patients with heart disease had higher Lp(a) levels than those who were free from heart disease.

As previously noted, a diet high in saturated fat lowers Lp(a) levels *(see papers 24, 70).*

Paper 86
Low fat/high carbohydrate diets implicated in heart disease

Weintraub MS et al Clearance of chylomicron remnants in normolipidaemic patients with coronary artery disease: case control study over three years.
British Medical Journal. 13 April 1996; 312 : 935

Chylomicrons are small fat globules composed of protein and fat. Chylomicrons are found in the blood and lymphatic fluid where they serve to transport fat from the intestines to other locations in the body. Chylomicron remnants are the chylomicrons after their transported fat has been "off-loaded".

The objective of this Israeli study was to test the hypothesis that subjects who clear chylomicron remnants slowly from the bloodstream may be at higher risk of heart disease than is indicated by their fasting blood fat and cholesterol levels. The trial lasted three years and included 85 men with coronary artery disease and 85 men with normal coronary arteries.

- The study head, Dr Moshe Weintraub, found that patients with heart disease had significantly higher concentrations of chylomicron remnants in the bloodstream than subjects without heart disease, even though both groups had normal cholesterol levels.

High concentrations of chylomicron remnants are caused by low fat/high carbohydrate diets *(see paper 65).*

Paper 87
Small dense LDL cholesterol
associated with heart disease in men

Lamarche B et al Small, Dense Low-Density Lipoprotein Particles as a Predictor of the Risk of Ischemic Heart Disease in Men. *Circulation.* 1997; 95 : 69-75

The lead researcher in this study, Dr Benoît Lamarche, is an Associate Professor in the Department of Food and Nutrition Sciences at Université Laval. His main area of interest is nutrition and its impact on cardiovascular health.

In this study, low-density lipoprotein cholesterol (LDL) diameter size was measured in 103 male patients with ischemic heart disease and 103 healthy control subjects to ascertain if LDL size is associated with ischemic heart disease.

- Dr Lamarche found that those men with the smallest diameter LDL had a 3.6-fold increase in the risk of ischemic heart disease compared with those with the largest diameter LDL.
- The study suggests that the presence of small, dense LDL particles may be associated with an increased risk of subsequently developing heart disease in men.

Consequently if LDL cholesterol particles are only associated with heart disease if they are of a small diameter, then large diameter LDL cholesterol does not have any association with heart disease.

Low fat/high carbohydrate diets can trigger small dense LDL cholesterol *(see paper 70)*.

Paper 88
High Triglyceride levels are
associated with heart disease

Gaziano JM et al Fasting Triglycerides, High-Density
Lipoprotein, and Risk of Myocardial Infarction.
Circulation. 1997; 96 : 2520-2525

Triglycerides are major components of very-low-density lipoprotein (VLDL) cholesterol and chylomicrons. A triglyceride consists of three molecules of fat combined with a molecule of the alcohol glycerol. Triglycerides come from the food we eat as well as from being produced by the body.

This study, from the *Harvard Medical School*, examined the inter-relationships of triglycerides and high-density lipoprotein cholesterol (HDL) with the risk of heart attack among 340 subjects (aged under 76) who had suffered a heart attack and an equal number of matched healthy control subjects.

The results of the study showed:

- Those with the highest triglycerides had almost seven times the risk of a heart attack compared to those with the lowest triglycerides.
- Those with the highest HDL cholesterol levels were somewhat protected from a heart attack compared to those with the lowest HDL cholesterol levels.

The paper demonstrated that a high triglyceride level is associated with heart disease. High triglyceride levels may be caused by carbohydrate consumption *(see papers 60, 62, 65, 69, 81).*

Another finding is that high HDL cholesterol levels appear to give protection from heart disease. A high fat diet raises HDL cholesterol levels *(see papers 21, 67).*

Paper 89
Apo B48, chylomicron
remnants and heart disease

Smith D et al Post-prandial chylomicron response may be predicted by a single measurement of plasma apolipoprotein

B48 in the fasting state. *European Journal of Clinical Investigation.* 1999 Mar; 29(3) : 204-9

Apolipoprotein B (apoB) is an apolipoprotein (protein) in chylomicrons and the primary apolipoprotein in low-density lipoprotein (LDL) cholesterol. There are two main types of apoB. ApoB48 is made in the small intestines and is associated with chylomicrons, whereas apoB100 is synthesized in the liver and is affiliated with LDL cholesterol.

The clearance from the bloodstream of chylomicron remnants was assessed in male subjects in this Australian study.

The study authors note that elevated levels of chylomicron remnants in the bloodstream are associated with heart disease.

• The study found that apoB48 concentration is a marker of chylomicron remnants. Therefore elevated apoB48 concentrations are associated with heart disease.

Low-fat/high-carbohydrate diets cause elevated levels of apoB48 (and apoB100) *(see papers 66, 70).*

Paper 90
Heart disease risk factors are increased
by a diet low in fat and high in carbohydrate

Sacks FM et al VLDL, Apolipoproteins B, CIII, and E, and Risk of Recurrent Coronary Events in the Cholesterol and Recurrent Events (CARE) Trial. *Circulation.* 2000; 102 : 1886

Very low-density lipoprotein (VLDL) cholesterol is a type of lipoprotein assembled by the liver from triglycerides, cholesterol, and apolipoproteins.

Apolipoprotein C-III (apoC-III) is the most abundant protein on chylomicrons and is a major component of the apolipoproteins in VLDL cholesterol.

In this five year study Frank Sacks, who is Professor of Cardiovascular Disease Prevention at the Harvard School of Public Health, measured the sizes of (i) VLDL–apolipoprotein (apo)B100, (ii) VLDL cholesterol and (iii) apoC-III in 418 patients who had either a heart attack or coronary death, and compared the measurements with those in 370 patients who did not have a cardiovascular event.

All factors, when elevated, (i)VLDL–apolipoprotein (apo)B100, (ii)VLDL cholesterol and (iii)apoC-III were associated with higher rates of heart disease.

All these elevated heart disease factors are associated with a diet low in fat and high in carbohydrate ie:

- VLDL–apolipoprotein (apo)B100 *(see paper 66)*
- VLDL cholesterol *(see paper 62)*
- apoC-III *(see paper 69)*

Paper 91
LDL cholesterol size: Small is bad
Berneisa K et al LDL size: does it matter?
Swiss Medical Weekly. 2004; 134 : 720-724

Dr Kaspar Berneisa reviewed the scientific evidence concerning LDL cholesterol size and disease.

He finds there are basically two different types of low-density lipoprotein cholesterol (LDL). These are classified as (good) pattern A, which are large and "fluffy" and (bad) pattern B which are small and "dense".

Dr Berneisa found that:

- Pattern B small dense LDL cholesterol has been accepted as a heart disease risk factor.
- Pattern B small dense LDL cholesterol are associated with a greater than two fold increased risk for developing type two diabetes.
- It has been shown that a very low fat, high carbohydrate diet can increase pattern B LDL cholesterol *(see paper 70)*.
- High fat diets are associated with an increase of pattern A large LDL cholesterol and a decrease of pattern B small dense LDL cholesterol *(see paper 30)*.

This paper demonstrates how pattern A LDL cholesterol, which are large and "fluffy" is relatively benign and pattern B LDL cholesterol which are small and "dense" is a known heart disease risk factor.

High fat diets promote the "good" pattern A, whereas low fat diets promote the "bad" pattern B.

Paper 92
Heart disease and stroke risk
increased by high carbohydrate diets

Ren J et al Relationship between serum non-high-density lipoprotein cholesterol and incidence of cardiovascular disease. *Zhonghua Xin Xue Guan Bing Za Zhi.* 2010 Oct; 38(10) : 934-8

The objective of this Chinese study, which lasted 12 years, was to evaluate the relationship between non high-density lipoprotein (non-HDL) cholesterol, very low-density lipoprotein (VLDL) cholesterol and heart disease and stroke in 29,937 Chinese aged 35-64 years.

- The study found that non-HDL is associated with increased risk of suffering heart disease and stroke and that VLDL plays a critical role in the development.

Non-HDL is comprised of low-density lipoprotein (LDL) cholesterol and VLDL. High levels of both LDL and VLDL are caused by high carbohydrate diets *(see papers 70, 62).*

The evidence from this chapter shows there may be more than one cause for the exponential rise in heart disease over the last century.

One of the reasons may be because of the increased use of pharmaceutical drugs which are prescribed supposedly to alleviate the rising problems of heart disease and obesity, but which in fact may exacerbate the problems.

Studies have shown that the ubiquitous aspirin in fact increase cardiovascular diseases by 23% and humble sleeping pills cause a 28% rise in heart attacks.

Soy is now now almost compulsory in many processed food products, whereas formerly it was relatively uncommon. Soy can also raise heart disease risk factors, thereby adding to the surge in heart disease rates.

Soy is part of the biggest change over the last 100 years or so, and that is the change in diet. There have been two other major changes.

The first change is the increase in highly processed, carbohydrate laden, low-fat foods.

This has happened because we have been encouraged by the powers that be to consume high carbohydrate, low-fat diets and as a result of this many food products are marketed as "low fat" or "low cholesterol."

This advice by the health authorities to eat less fat is working, because we are consuming less fat than even in the 1970s. In that time there has also been a sharp rise in carbohydrate consumption. Most of these carbohydrates are in the form of processed foods such as cornflakes, coco pops, pasta, pizza etc.

This low-fat fare has adversely affected our nutrient intake. Studies have revealed that low-fat diets will result in deficiencies of essential fats, minerals (such as zinc), the vitamins A,D,E and K and various hormones.

The second big change in diet is the big drop in the consumption of saturated animal fats (eg butter and lard) accompanied by a massive rise in margarine and vegetable oils such as sunflower oil, safflower oil and soy oil.

As a comparison; since 1909 the amount of butter consumed has declined by 360% whereas margarine intake has risen by 550%.

To sum up the changes in our diet, we now eat more soy, more processed carbohydrates, more vegetable oils and less saturated animal fats.

So what effect has this fundamental change in the food we eat had on our heart health?

High levels of the hormone *insulin*, the amino acid *homocysteine* and the protein *C-reactive protein* are linked to higher rates of heart disease. High-carbohydrate diets tend to promote the formation of these substances, whereas high-fat diets tend to lower them.

Chapter 3 demonstrated that elevated high-density lipoprotein (HDL) cholesterol levels are protective against heart disease. But what about the other types of cholesterol? And what exactly is cholesterol?

Cholesterol cannot actually flow around the blood on its own accord. It has to hitch a ride on molecules called lipoproteins to be able to circulate around the body. So when you hear people talking about cholesterol levels, they are actually describing lipoprotein levels.

These lipoproteins include; high-density lipoprotein (HDL) cholesterol, low-density lipoprotein (LDL) cholesterol, very low-density lipoprotein (VLDL) cholesterol, chylomicrons and lipoprotein (a).

In addition to cholesterol getting a free ride on these lipoproteins, molecules called triglycerides are integrated into VLDL cholesterol and chylomicrons and, (not surprisingly because of the name lipoprotein), proteins called apolipoproteins form part of the lipoproteins.

The evidence has demonstrated that the heart friendly HDL cholesterol and apolipoprotein A-1 levels are increased by a diet rich in saturated fat. Conversely a diet low in fat and high in carbohydrate will lower the levels of HDL cholesterol and apolipoprotein A-1.

LDL cholesterol may be considered either benign or dangerous depending on its particle size. Large LDL is benign whereas small LDL has been shown to be dangerous. Studies show that a high saturated fat consumption promotes the formation of benign large LDL, but high-carbohydrate diets stimulate the formation of the dangerous small LDL.

High levels of triglycerides, the apolipoproteins B & C, and the other types of cholesterol; VLDL, chylomicrons and lipoprotein (a) are all linked to higher rates of heart disease. Scientific papers reveal that a high saturated fat diet will lower the unhealthy high levels of these substances, whilst a diet high in carbohydrate will increase the unhealthy levels even further.

So the evidence has demonstrated that high carbohydrate, low fat diets will promote unhealthy levels of various substances, but what does this mean for the actual health of people?

Papers have revealed that high carbohydrate diets will lead to more blocked arteries.

In another paper, a 10-year study showed that a high consumption of carbohydrates was accompanied by a rise of up to 98% in heart disease.

Another massive study of over one million men delivered the news that the men on a low fat, vegetable based diet had a seven fold increased risk of heart disease compared to the men on a diet that provided 19 times more fat.

So this evidence has revealed that a high carbohydrate diet promotes heart disease and a high saturated fat diet is heart healthy.

Now about this other big change in the diet; namely how the reduction in saturated fat has been combined with an enormous rise in vegetable oils and margarine. What are the health consequences?

In studies comparing the health effects of butter with margarine, the data shows that margarine promotes higher levels of the (bad) triglycerides and (bad) chylomicrons.

Margarine also decreases the levels of the heart healthy HDL cholesterol and apolipoprotein A-1.

Other unwanted effects of margarine include making the blood flow sluggishly and damaging the lining of the blood vessels.

Papers that measure margarine consumption find that high consumption leads to an increase in heart disease.

With margarine production been a massive scale industrial process, made with cheap oils and a myriad of additives and preservatives, it's not surprising margarine elevates heart disease rates.

To answer the questions from the start of the chapter:

What then are we doing different from a time when there was very little heart disease, to the present day when it seems heart disease is almost compulsory?
   We used to eat whole real food with natural fats.

We now eat; genetically modified, highly processed, low-fat, added sugar, laden with industrially produced rancid vegetable oil, additives and preservatives commodities.

Are we told the correct dietary advice?
   We are told animal protein and animal fat will lead to heart disease. So we are advised to eat a low-fat, high carbohydrate diet and to only use vegetable oils.

The scientific evidence shows this official dietary advice is completely misguided, and despite all the medical knowledge and modern facilities at our disposal, heart disease incidence has exploded since the early 1900s.

So what do the experts say?

The next chapter reveals the thoughts of eminent professors and doctors.

CHAPTER 5

Comment by eminent professors and doctors

This chapter includes contributions from professors and doctors, who are leading experts on the subject of cardiovascular disease.

Paper 93
Doctor says: The Diet/Heart Hypothesis is the greatest deception of our times

Mann G Coronary Heart Disease - "Doing the Wrong Things".
Nutrition Today. July/August 1985;
Volume 20 Issue 4 pg 12-15

Dr George V Mann is a Johns Hopkins-educated biochemist and physician and was on the faculty of Vanderbilt University in Nashville.

Mann reviewed the literature concerning the Diet/Heart Hypothesis.

After examining the evidence Mann found:

- The advice to replace saturated animal fat with polyunsaturated vegetable oils and restricting eggs, was a presumptuous guess because there was no supporting data to show either the safety of efficacy of such dietary strategy.

- Many long and expensive trials have since been designed to show evidence for the safety and efficacy of such dietary strategy. All those trials have failed.
- Dietary restriction of cholesterol has NOT been shown to be an effective way to lower high cholesterol.
- Substitution of saturated fat in the diet with polyunsaturated fat has produced ominous signs of toxicity, often manifested by increased rates of cancer.
- 93% of the population and the majority of physicians believe saturated fat and cholesterol are the "bad guys". The Diet/Heart Hypothesis is a propaganda success of Goebbelsian proportions.
- Clinical trials of the Diet/Heart Hypothesis have cost billions of dollars. Never in the history of science have so many costly experiments failed so consistently.

Dr Mann states: *"A generation of citizens has grown up since the Diet/Heart Hypothesis was launched as official dogma. They have been misled by the greatest deception of our times, the notion that consumption of animal fat causes heart disease."*

Paper 94
Doctor condemns
the campaign against cholesterol

Stare FJ The AMA's Campaign Against Cholesterol. *Journal of the American Medical Association.* 1989; 261(22) : 3240-3241

Dr Stare was an emeritus professor of nutrition and the founding chairman of the department of nutrition at the Harvard School of Public Health.

Dr Stare states: *"The cholesterol factor is of minor importance as a risk factor in cardiovascular disease. Of far more importance are smoking, hypertension, obesity, diabetes, insufficient physical activity and stress".*

He also added *"The National Cholesterol Education Program was most unfortunate, because it gives undue emphasis to a minor risk factor in cardiovascular disease and thus false hope to millions of individuals".*

Paper 95
Director of the world's longest running heart study says those that eat more cholesterol and fat - weigh the least and are more physically active

Castelli WP Concerning the Possibility of a Nut...
Archives of Internal Medicine. 1992; 152(7) : 1371-1372

The Framingham Heart Study is a long-term, ongoing cardiovascular study on residents of the town of Framingham, Massachusetts. It is the world's longest running heart disease study and began in 1948 with 5,209 adult subjects from Framingham, and is now on its third generation of participants.

Dr William Castelli, a director of the Framingham Heart Study, declared: *"In Framingham, Mass. we found that the people who ate the most cholesterol, ate the most saturated fat, ate the most calories, weighed the least, and were the most physically active."*

Paper 96
Professor finds that the knowledge of the factors causing heart disease is based on unscientific methodology and therefore the lipid hypothesis is invalid

Stehbens WE Science, atherosclerosis and
the "age of unreason": a review. *Integrative
Physiological and Behavioural Science.*
1993 Oct-Dec; 28(4) : 388-95

Professor William Stehbens was the founding professor and the chairman of the pathology department at the Wellington School of Medicine.

Professor Stehbens reports that research into the build up of plaque in the arteries has been dominated by the lipid hypothesis. He continues that the pathology of both the cholesterol-fed animal and of familial hypercholesterolemia has been misrepresented and that the vascular lesions of these disorders are not a build up of plaque but manifestations of fat storage.

Professor Stehbens finds there are fundamental defects in the epidemiological approach to the causes of the build up of plaque and these include:

- Misuse of the cause and risk factors.
- Misuse of coronary heart disease as an imprecise and inappropriate surrogate endpoint in clinical and mortality studies.

- Use of fallacious causes of death on death certificates and mortality rates.
- Mistaken assumed causal role of risk factors.
- Use of misleading dietary data.
- Ecological fallacies.
- Misrepresentation of statistical correlations and selection bias.
- Failure to take note of inconsistencies.
- Inappropriate use of the blood cholesterol level as a surrogate of plaque build up (substitution game) without demonstration of any such effect on arteries.
- Wrong conclusions concerning pathological and experimental corroborative evidence.

Professor Stehbens concludes; *"the epidemiology of the build up of plaque is based on unscientific methodology and the lipid hypothesis as currently envisaged is invalid. There is need to review the cholesterol-lowering campaign especially for people with normal cholesterol levels."*

Paper 97
Doctor says: Contrary to a widespread opinion, cholesterol lowering does not appear to be a very effective way of reducing cardiac and overall mortality in the general population

de Lorgeril M Cholesterol lowering
and mortality: time for a new paradigm?
Nutrition, Metabolism and Cardiovascular Diseases. 2006 Sep; 16(6) : 387-90

Dr Michel de Lorgeril holds positions at Joseph Fourier University and the National Centre of Scientific Research in Grenoble, France and is internationally known for his work on cardiovascular disease.

Dr de Lorgeril states: *"Careful analysis of the available data, including randomised trials, indicates that, contrary to a widespread opinion, cholesterol lowering does not appear to be a very effective way of reducing cardiac and overall mortality in the general population"*.

Paper 98
End of the road for the diet-heart theory?
Werko L End of the road for the diet-heart theory?
Scandinavian Cardiovascular Journal. 2008 May 9 : 1-6

Dr Lars Werko is a leading cardiologist in Sweden.

In this review Dr Werko describes how the diet-heart theory is flawed. He points out that:

- Having a heart attack is NOT synonymous with clogged arteries.
- Shenanigans with the data has been used to obscure the negative results of randomised multi-factorial trials.
- Side effects of the statin group of medicines have been more or less neglected in the large amount of clinical trials.

Paper 99
Professor says the adverse effects of the cholesterol campaign on health, quality of life, the economy and medical research are inestimable

Rosch PJ Cholesterol does not cause coronary heart disease in contrast to stress. *Scandinavian Cardiovascular Journal.* 2008 Aug; 42(4) : 244-9

Paul Rosch, MD, is a clinical professor of medicine and psychiatry at New York Medical College.

Professor Rosch reviewed the evidence on cholesterol and heart disease.

He found:

- The belief that heart disease is due to high cholesterol from increased saturated fat intake originated from experiments in herbivorous animals. This belief was built on by evidence that apparently confirmed the hypothesis, but which ignored contradictory data.
- The idea has been perpetuated by powerful forces for the preservation of profit margins.
- Opponents of the hypothesis find it difficult to publish their scientifically supported opinions.
- The advent of statins has further fuelled this fallacious lipid hypothesis, despite hard evidence that their effect is not due to the lowering of cholesterol levels and that serious side effects have been repressed and alleged benefits have been exaggerated.

Professor Rosch concludes; *"the adverse effects of the cholesterol campaign on health, quality of life, the economy and medical research are inestimable. It is imperative that public health officials, physicians and patients are apprised of proof that it is misguided, malicious and malignant."*

Paper 100
The cholesterol campaign should be revised by scientists without links to the food or drug industry

Ravnskov U Hypercholesterolaemia: Should medical science ignore the past? *British Medical Journal.* 2008; 337 : a1681

Dr Uffe Ravnskov is a Swedish physician and cholesterol expert. He has published more than 100 papers and letters critical of the cholesterol campaign; most of them in major medical journals.

Dr Ravnskov makes the following observations:

- No association between cholesterol and degree of plaque build up has been found in post mortem studies ofunselected individuals.
- High cholesterol levels are not risk factors for patients with renal failure, diabetic patients, women, or old people.
- Old people with high cholesterol levels live longer than those with low cholesterol levels.
- In cohorts of people with familial hypercholestero laemia (genetically high cholesterol), cholesterol is not associated with any increase in the incidence or prevalence of heart disease, and their average life span is similar to the rest of the population.
- Heart disease rates or total death rates have never been reduced in any randomised, controlled, uni-factorial, dietary, cholesterol lowering trial.
- No clinical trial or X-ray examination of the blood vessels has found a connection between individual degree of cholesterol lowering and outcome.

- More than 20 studies have found that patients with heart disease ate the same amount of saturated fat as did healthy individuals.
- Saturated fat intake, is similar or lower in patients with heart disease compared with healthy controls in five case-control studies.
- The effect of statin treatment is highly exaggerated and is not due to cholesterol lowering. Only a small percentage of the population might benefit - and then only if they are men at high risk - and the benefit is easily surpassed by the side effects that are more frequent and more serious than reported in the trials of statin drugs, if reported at all.

Dr Ravnskov concludes: *"Revision of the cholesterol campaign by scientists without links to the food or drug industry seems urgent."*

Paper 101
Professor says the cholesterol
6hypothesis is false and should be buried

Schersten T The cholesterol hypothesis: time for the obituary?
Scandinavian Cardiovascual Journal. 2011 Dec; 45(6) : 322-3

Dr Schersten is a professor of Vascular Surgery, University of Göteborg and was previously Principal Secretary of the Swedish Medical Research Council.

Professor Schersten finds that the cholesterol hypothesis that links cholesterol intake and blood cholesterol levels to cardiovascular disease has little or no scientific backing that is relevant for the human species.

He concludes that the hypothesis is false and should be buried.

––––––––––––

The consensus amongst these experts is that the diet/heart hypothesis was based on flawed studies, and then perpetuated by fallacious data.

They find that clinical trials, costing billions of dollars, which were conceived to prove the hypothesis, have failed miserably.

No dietary, cholesterol-lowering trial has ever succeeded in lowering the rates of coronary deaths or total deaths.

They describe the notion that consumption of animal fat causes heart disease is the greatest medical deception of our times.

Their research concludes there is no scientific backing for the diet/heart hypothesis and it should be buried.

CHAPTER 6

Summary of the evidence

The scientific evidence has revealed the saturated fat/cholesterol/heart disease hypothesis is based on irrelevant studies conducted on herbivorous animals and out of date and deeply flawed studies in the 1950s.

Saturated fat and dietary cholesterol have been shown to actually reduce heart disease rates, whilst low-fat/high carbohydrate based diets promote heart problems. The rise in consumption of vegetable oils is also implicated in fuelling heart disease.

High blood cholesterol levels are not a factor in heart disease, and in fact high cholesterol levels are associated with a longer lifespan.

Eminent professors and doctors comment that the diet/heart hypothesis is based on unscientific evidence and that the adverse effects of the hypothesis on health, quality of life, the economy and medical research are inestimable.

Dr George Mann, a distinguished physician, comments "The diet/heart hypothesis is a propaganda success of Goebbelsian proportions."

This review of the scientific literature demonstrates:

- ❖ High blood cholesterol levels are associated with a longer life.
- ❖ Diets low in fat and high in carbohydrate promote heart disease.
- ❖ Polyunsaturated vegetable oils promote heart disease.
- ❖ Diets high in cholesterol and saturated fat prevent heart disease.

Appendix 1

Glossary

Apolipoproteins
proteins that bind fat and cholesterol to form lipoproteins.

Apolipoprotein A-I (apoA-1)
the major protein component of high density
lipoprotein (HDL).

Apolipoprotein B48 (apoB48)
a unique protein to chylomicrons from the small intestine.

Apolipoprotein B100 (apoB100)
a protein found in lipoproteins originating from the
liver such as very low density lipoprotein (VLDL) and
low density lipoproteins (LDL).

Apolipoprotein C-III (apoC-III)
a protein component of very low density lipoprotein
(VLDL).

Atherosclerosis
a disease in which plaque builds up inside your arteries.

Cardiovascular disease
a class of diseases that involve the heart or blood vessels
such as heart disease and stroke.

Case control study
are usually but not exclusively retrospective studies.

Cholesterol
a waxy substance found in your body that is needed to produce hormones, vitamin D and bile. Cholesterol is also important for protecting nerves and for the structure of cells.

Chylomicrons
carries triglycerides from the intestines to the liver, to skeletal muscle, and to adipose tissue.

Cohort studies
are usually but not exclusively prospective studies.

Control group
the people that do not receive the treatment being studied.

Coronary heart disease
the narrowing or blockage of the coronary arteries.

C-reactive protein (CRP)
a protein found in the blood, the levels of which rise in response to inflammation.

Diet-heart hypothesis
is the idea that dietary saturated fat and dietary cholesterol, raise blood cholesterol and therefore contribute to the risk of heart disease.

Endocrinologist
a doctor who specializes in treating disorders of the endocrine system (hormones), such as diabetes, certain cancers and many other diseases.

Endothelial dysfunction
a condition in which the endothelium (inner lining) of blood vessels does not function normally.

Epidemiological study
the study of health-events, health-characteristics or health-determinant patterns in a population.

Familial hypercholesterolemia
a genetic disorder characterized by high cholesterol levels.

Fatty acid
a saturated, monounsaturated or polyunsaturated fat.

Glycemic index
a measure of the effects of carbohydrates on blood sugar levels.

Glycemic load
a ranking system for carbohydrate content in food portions based on their glycemic index and a standardised portion size of 100g.

High density lipoproteins (HDL)
collects cholesterol from the body's tissues, and bring it back to the liver.

High density lipoprotein 2 (HDL2)
a type of high density lipoprotein (HDL).

Hispanics
are Americans with origins in the Hispanic countries of Latin America or in Spain.

Homocysteine
a non-protein amino acid.

Inflammation
inflammation of the arteries is linked to heart disease.

Insulin
a hormone secreted from the pancreas that removes excess glucose from the blood.

Ischaemic (or ischemic) heart disease
a disease characterised by reduced blood supply to the heart.

Lipid Hypothesis
proposes a connection between cholesterol levels and the development of heart disease.

Lipoprotein
a molecule containing protein, fat and cholesterol that circulates around the bloodstream.

Lipoprotein (a) [(Lp(a)]
a type of lipoprotein. High Lp(a) in blood is a risk factor for heart disease and stroke.

Lipoprotein A-1
a type of high density lipoprotein (HDL).

Lipoprotein A-1:A-2
a type of high density lipoprotein (HDL).

Low density lipoproteins (LDL)
carries cholesterol from the liver to cells of the body.

Macronutrients
fat, protein or carbohydrate.

Monounsaturated fat
a fat that has 2 hydrogen atoms missing which are replaced with one double bond.

Mortality rate
a measure of the number of deaths.

Multi-factorial study
experimental investigation of the simultaneous influence of several variables.

Pediatrics
the branch of medicine that deals with the care of infants and children and the treatment of their diseases.

Placebo
an inactive substance administered to a patient usually to compare its effects with those of a real treatment.

Polyunsaturated fat
a fat that has 4 or more hydrogen atoms missing which are replaced with two or more double bonds. A very unstable fat that goes rancid easily.

Prospective study
watches for outcomes, such as the development of a disease, during the study period and relates this to other factors such as suspected risk or protection factors.

Reactive hypoglycemia
low blood sugar that occurs after a meal-usually one to three hours after eating.

Retrospective study
looks backwards and examines exposures to suspected risk or protection factors in relation to an outcome that is established at the start of the study.

Saturated fat
a fat that has its full complement of hydrogen atoms. A very stable fat that is good for cooking with.

Statins
are a class of drugs used to lower cholesterol levels. They have many adverse side effects.

Trans fat
man made artificial fat. The consumption of trans fats increases the risk of coronary heart disease.

Triglycerides
the major form of fat stored by the body. A triglyceride consists of three molecules of fat combined with a molecule of the alcohol glycerol.

Very low density lipoproteins (VLDL)
carries (newly synthesized) triglycerides from the liver to adipose tissue.

Appendix 2

Further resources

Websites:

www.thincs.org

The International Network of Cholesterol Sceptics (or THINCS) is a group of scientists, physicians, and other academicians from around the world who dispute the widely accepted saturated fat/cholesterol causes heart disease hypothesis. THINCS was founded in January 2003.

www.dietsandscience.com

I've run this website since 2010. I write easy to read reviews on over 850 diet, lifestyle & health studies from research centres, universities and peer reviewed journals.

Books:

Put your heart in your mouth by Natasha Campbell-McBride

The great cholesterol con by Anthony Colpo

Fat and cholesterol are good for you by Uffe Ravnskov

Nutrition and physical degeneration by Weston A Price

Appendix 3

List of studies

Chapter 1: It's never been proved that high cholesterol causes heart disease

1 Rabbits and cholesterol
2 Ancel Keys 6 countries study actually shows the more animal fat and animal protein you eat, the longer you live!
3 If he'd wanted, Ancel Keys could have proved that saturated fat gives protection from heart disease
4 Harvard pathologist finds that high blood cholesterol is NOT the cause of blocked arteries
5 Research team reveal cholesterol levels have NO correlation with clogged arteries
6 The cholesterol/heart disease hypothesis is false
7 Analysis of 1,700 patients finds NO association between the level of cholesterol in the blood and the incidence of heart disease
8 Another study finds that cholesterol levels are NOT connected to clogged arteries

Chapter 2: Dietary cholesterol and saturated fat lower the rates of heart disease

9 An increase in dietary fat and cholesterol is associated with less heart disease

10 As saturated fat and cholesterol increase in the diet, then rates of heart attack and death decrease

11 Dietary cholesterol does NOT increase the risk of developing clogged arteries in pre-menopausal women

12 Diets high in cholesterol and saturated fat lower the risk of heart disease and diabetes

13 High cholesterol diet results in LESS heart disease risk for men and women

14 Vegetarians have a higher risk of heart disease compared to meat eaters

15 Dietary cholesterol in eggs gives multiple health benefits

16 A review of recent scientific data clearly demonstrates that dietary cholesterol is NOT correlated with increased risk for heart disease

17 Dietary fat is not responsible for heart disease

18 Restriction of saturated fat leads to higher rates of heart disease

19 High saturated fat diets are associated with virtually NO heart disease

20 Saturated fat consumption improves beneficial HDL cholesterol levels

21 Analysis of 27 trials finds the best way to raise HDL (good cholesterol) is to eat saturated fat

22 Increased saturated fat consumption leads to lower rates of heart disease and stroke

23 Men who eat the most saturated fat have a 27% DECREASE in heart disease deaths

24 Saturated fat lowers (bad) Lp(a) cholesterol levels

25 Increasing dietary saturated fat may help you to live longer

26 High animal protein intake associated with a lower risk of heart disease for women

27 Saturated fat helps to reduce heart disease risk factors

Chapter 3: High cholesterol levels help you live longer

44 Cholesterol levels have no influence on heart disease or mortality

45 Low cholesterol is associated with marked increase in mortality in heart failure

46 In patients with chronic heart failure, lower total cholesterol levels are associated with earlier death

47 Low cholesterol levels are strongly associated with increased mortality in patients with nonischemic, systolic heart failure

48 High cholesterol is a marker for longevity

49 For each 1-mmol/L (38mg/dL) decrease in cholesterol levels, heart failure patients have a 26% increase in mortality risk

50 A 10ml INCREASE in cholesterol levels are associated with a 4% DECREASED risk of mortality from heart failure

51 Low cholesterol levels are associated with higher death rates in stroke, heart failure, and cancer

52 High cholesterol levels are associated with a 22% DECREASE in stroke incidence

53 The higher your cholesterol levels - the longer you live!

54 High HDL cholesterol gives protection from heart attacks

55 Association of low levels of HDL and HDL2 cholesterol with heart disease

56 Low HDL cholesterol and increased heart disease

57 Low HDL cholesterol increases coronary heart disease death in the elderly

58 The "bad" low-density lipoprotein (LDL) cholesterol levels have NO association with heart disease rates

59 Saturated fat can help to lower the rates of heart disease

Chapter 4: What does cause heart disease?

60 High carbohydrate diets are associated with an increase in incidence of coronary artery disease

61 Study of over 1 Million men shows that eating a low-fat, vegetable based diet gives a 7-fold increased risk of heart disease

62 High carbohydrate diet leads to adverse health effects

63 Diets high in carbohydrates which have a high glycemic load, increase heart disease risk by 98%

64 Low fat diets in children may lead to clogged arteries in adulthood

65 Low fat/high carbohydrate diets are associated with higher heart disease risk

66 Heart disease risk is increased by a high carbohydrate diet

67 Low fat diets do not provide adequate nutrition and increase heart disease risk factors

68 In postmenopausal women, carbohydrate intake is associated with a progression of heart disease

69 Low fat, high carbohydrate diets increase the risk of heart disease

70 Increase in heart disease risk factors on a low fat high carbohydrate diet

71 Vegetable oils implicated in increased death rates

72 Margarine increases the risk of heart disease

73 Medium or high intake of margarine is associated with a 50% increased risk of a non-fatal heart attack

74 Margarine intake increases the risk of heart disease

75 Margarine damages the lining of blood vessels

76 Sunflower oil and olive oil increase heart disease risk factors compared to butter

77 Sunflower oil damages the blood vessels

78 High insulin levels linked to heart disease

79 Vegan diet may lead to heart disease risk

80 Soy consumption increases Lp(a), an independent risk factor for heart disease

81 High fat diets reduce dangerous C-reactive protein levels by 52.6%

82 Aspirin increases the risk of heart disease and stroke

83 Appetite suppressant pills lead to a 28% higher risk of having a heart attack and a 36% higher risk of developing a stroke

84 A high saturated fat diet gives protection from heart disease

85 High Lp(a) levels linked to heart disease - Saturated fat lowers Lp(a) levels

86 Low fat/high carbohydrate diets implicated in heart disease

87 Small dense LDL cholesterol associated with heart disease in men

88 High Triglyceride levels are associated with heart disease

89 Apo B48, chylomicron remnants and heart disease

90 Heart disease risk factors are increased by a diet low in fat and high in carbohydrate

91 LDL cholesterol size: Small is bad

92 Heart disease and stroke risk increased by high carbohydrate diets

Chapter 5: Comment by eminent professors and doctors

93 Doctor says: The Diet/Heart Hypothesis is the greatest deception of our times

94 Doctor condemns the campaign against cholesterol

95 Director of the world's longest running heart study says those that eat more cholesterol and fat-weigh the least and are more physically active

96 Professor finds that the knowledge of the factors causing heart disease is based on unscientific methodology and therefore the lipid hypothesis is invalid

Index

(Refers to paper numbers)